THE 30 MINUTES Diabetic RENAL DIET COOKBOOK FOR BEGINNERS

By

Jane F Garraway

Copyright © 2024

TABLE OF CONTENTS

SCAN HERE TO CHECK OUT OTHER BOOKS BY JANE GARRAWAY

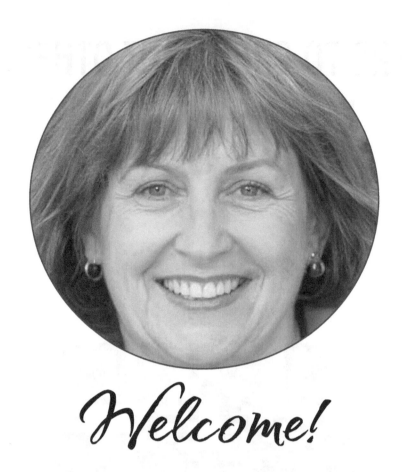

Welcome!

I am thrilled to have you purchase this cookbook. Whether you are an experienced home cook or just starting out, my collection of recipes is always designed to inspire and my goal is to make cooking an enjoyable and healthy experience for everyone.

Within these pages, you'll find a diverse range of dishes, each crafted with love and attention to detail.

Cooking is not just about preparing food; it's about creating memories, exploring new flavors, and sharing delicious and healthy meals with your loved ones. I encourage you to experiment, make these recipes your own, and savor every moment of the process.

Thank you for allowing me to be a part of your journey. Let's get cooking!

Jane Garraway

UNDERSTANDING CHRONIC KIDNEY DISEASE (CKD)

A diagnosis of Chronic Kidney Disease (CKD) indicates that your kidneys are not functioning at their best. CKD progresses through various stages, each reflecting a different level of kidney function. Understanding your specific stage, the underlying causes, and potential treatment options is crucial. Think of your healthcare providers as your dedicated coaches, guiding you through a strategic plan to protect your kidney health. This plan might include specific medications, dietary changes, and regular health check-ups. Just as mastering a sport requires learning the rules and strategies, gaining a thorough understanding of CKD empowers you to manage your condition effectively and maintain your well-being.

THE ESSENTIAL ROLES OF THE KIDNEYS

The kidneys are vital organs that play a crucial role in maintaining your overall health. Here's a look at their primary functions:

1. **Blood Filtration:** The kidneys filter your blood, removing waste products, toxins, and excess substances like urea, creatinine, and electrolytes.

2. **Fluid Balance:** They regulate the balance of fluids in your body, controlling the retention or excretion of water and electrolytes such as sodium, potassium, and calcium.

3. **Blood Pressure Regulation:** The kidneys help regulate blood pressure by managing fluid volume in blood vessels and releasing hormones that influence blood vessel constriction.

4. **Red Blood Cell Production:** They produce erythropoietin (EPO), a hormone that stimulates the bone marrow to produce red blood cells, which carry oxygen throughout your body.

5. **Acid-Base Balance:** The kidneys maintain a stable pH balance in your body by excreting excess acids or bases, which is essential for enzyme function and chemical reactions.

6. **Vitamin D Activation:** By activating vitamin D, the kidneys support bone health and regulate calcium and phosphorus levels.

7. **Hormone Regulation:** The kidneys release hormones that govern various bodily functions, including blood pressure regulation, red blood cell production, and calcium metabolism.

8. **Waste Elimination:** The kidneys filter waste products from your bloodstream, ensuring these harmful substances are excreted in urine.

In short, the kidneys are indispensable for maintaining a balanced internal environment, regulating blood pressure, and contributing to your overall health.

EXPLORING CHRONIC KIDNEY DISEASE (CKD)

Chronic Kidney Disease (CKD) is characterized by a gradual loss of kidney function over time. The kidneys, which serve as the body's filtration system, become less efficient due to factors such as high blood pressure, diabetes, or other health conditions.

MANAGING CKD EFFECTIVELY

Your healthcare team, including nephrologists and dietitians, will work together to create a personalized CKD management plan. This plan may include medications, dietary guidance, and regular health assessments.

A. **Healthy Eating:** Following a specialized diet that is low in sodium, certain fruits, and specific foods can reduce the strain on your kidneys, slow CKD progression, and enhance your overall health.

B. **Blood Pressure Control:** Keeping your blood pressure within a healthy range is crucial. Your healthcare providers may recommend medications and lifestyle changes to achieve this.

C. **Blood Sugar Control:** If you have diabetes, managing your blood sugar is essential to prevent further kidney damage.

D. **Staying Active:** Regular exercise benefits your kidneys and overall health. Always consult your healthcare provider before starting a new exercise regimen.

E. **Hydration:** Maintaining balanced fluid intake is important. Your healthcare team will advise you on the appropriate amount to support optimal kidney function.

F. **Medications:** It's vital to take prescribed medications as directed. Some medications may need adjustment due to CKD.

G. **Quit Smoking & Limit Alcohol:** Smoking and excessive alcohol intake can harm your kidneys. Quitting smoking and moderating alcohol consumption are important steps.

THE STAGES OF CKD

CKD progresses through five stages, each representing a different level of kidney function:

→**Stage 1:** Mild kidney damage, often without noticeable symptoms.

→**Stage 2:** Mild decrease in kidney function, still with few symptoms.

→**Stage 3:** Moderate decline in kidney function, with potential symptoms.

→**Stage 4:** Severe decline in kidney function, with more pronounced symptoms and health complications.

→**Stage 5:** Kidney failure, requiring dialysis or a transplant to sustain life.

CAUSES OF CHRONIC KIDNEY DISEASE (CKD)

CKD can be caused by various factors that gradually impair kidney function over time. Common causes include:

1. **Diabetes:** High blood sugar can damage blood vessels and kidney structures, leading to decreased function.

2. **High Blood Pressure (Hypertension):** Prolonged high blood pressure can strain kidney blood vessels, causing gradual damage.

3. **Glomerulonephritis:** Inflammation and damage to the kidney's filtering units (glomeruli).

4. **Polycystic Kidney Disease (PKD):** An inherited disorder causing cyst growth within the kidneys, hindering function.

5. **Obstructed Urinary Tract:** Conditions like kidney stones or tumors can block urine flow, damaging the kidneys.

6. **Recurrent Kidney Infections:** Repeated infections can scar the kidneys and contribute to CKD.

7. **Autoimmune Diseases:** Conditions like lupus can cause the immune system to attack the kidneys.

8. **Excessive Use of Pain Relievers:** Long-term use of non-prescription pain relievers like ibuprofen can harm the kidneys.

9. **Exposure to Toxins:** Prolonged exposure to certain toxins can damage the kidneys.

10. **Aging:** Natural decline in kidney function with age increases CKD risk.

11. **Cardiovascular Disease:** Heart conditions can affect blood flow to the kidneys, contributing to CKD.

Managing these underlying causes and risk factors is key to preventing or slowing CKD progression.

SLOWING DOWN CKD PROGRESSION

Slowing CKD progression requires a holistic approach, involving lifestyle changes, medications, and consistent medical care. Here are strategies to help:

1. **Control Blood Pressure:** Work with your healthcare provider to maintain healthy blood pressure through medication, diet, exercise, and stress management.

2. **Manage Blood Sugar:** If you have diabetes, effective blood sugar management is crucial. Follow your diabetes management plan and monitor levels regularly.

3. **Adopt a Kidney-Friendly Diet:** Consult a registered dietitian to create a low-sodium, low-phosphorus, and low-potassium diet. Focus on lean proteins, whole grains, and a variety of fruits and vegetables.

4. **Limit Protein Intake:** Too much protein can strain your kidneys. Moderation, especially with animal proteins, helps preserve kidney function.

5. **Monitor Fluid Intake:** Follow your healthcare provider's advice on fluid intake to maintain balance, avoiding both overhydration and dehydration.

6. **Quit Smoking:** Smoking damages blood vessels and can worsen kidney damage. Quitting supports overall health and kidney function.

7. **Exercise Regularly:** Physical activity helps control blood pressure, manage blood sugar, and maintain a healthy weight. Consult your healthcare provider before starting a new exercise routine.

8. **Take Medications as Prescribed:** Follow your healthcare provider's instructions for medications that manage blood pressure, blood sugar, or other related conditions.

9. **Stay Hydrated Safely:** Adhere to fluid intake recommendations to avoid dehydration or overhydration.

10. **Avoid Nephrotoxic Substances:** Be cautious with over-the-counter medications and supplements, as some may harm your kidneys. Always consult your healthcare provider before taking new medications.

11. **Manage Stress:** Chronic stress can negatively impact your health. Practice relaxation techniques like meditation or stress-reducing activities.

12. **Regular Medical Check-Ups:** Keep up with appointments and recommended lab tests to monitor kidney function, blood pressure, and overall health.

Slowing CKD progression requires dedication and close collaboration with your healthcare team. They will provide personalized guidance and adapt strategies based on your unique needs.

FOOD LIST FOR OPTIMAL RENAL HEALTH

Here's a guide to low-sodium, low-potassium, and important foods to consider for improving your renal health:

LOW-SODIUM FOODS

- **Fresh Fruits:** Apples, berries (blueberries, strawberries, raspberries), peaches, pears (limit portions for potassium).
- **Fresh Vegetables:** Cauliflower, bell peppers, zucchini, green beans, carrots.
- **Lean Proteins:** Skinless poultry, lean cuts of beef or pork, fish (rinse canned fish to reduce sodium).
- **Whole Grains:** Brown rice, whole wheat pasta, quinoa, oats.
- **Dairy and Alternatives:** Low-sodium or sodium-free milk, yogurt, and cheese.
- **Nuts and Seeds:** Unsalted almonds, walnuts, chia seeds.
- **Legumes:** Lentils, chickpeas, beans (rinse canned beans to reduce sodium).
- **Herbs and Spices:** Flavor meals with herbs and spices instead of salt.
- **Healthy Fats:** Olive oil, avocado.

LOW-POTASSIUM FOODS

- **Fruits:** Apples, berries, peaches, pears, plums.
- **Vegetables:** Cauliflower, bell peppers, zucchini, green beans, carrots, lettuce.
- **Grains:** White rice, white pasta.
- **Proteins:** Skinless poultry, lean cuts of beef or pork, fish (in moderation).
- **Dairy and Alternatives:** Low-potassium milk, yogurt, and cheese.
- **Beverages:** Most clear sodas, apple juice, cranberry juice (in moderation).

IMPORTANT FOODS FOR RENAL HEALTH

- **Omega-3 Fatty Acids:** Fatty fish such as salmon, mackerel, and sardines are excellent sources of omega-3 fatty acids, which have anti-inflammatory properties that can benefit kidney health. For those avoiding fish, flaxseeds, chia seeds, and walnuts offer plant-based alternatives.

- **Antioxidant-Rich Fruits and Vegetables:** Blueberries, red grapes, and strawberries are high in antioxidants, which can protect kidney cells from oxidative stress. Additionally, cruciferous vegetables like cauliflower and cabbage are packed with vitamins and fiber while being low in potassium.

- **Whole Grains:** Whole grains such as brown rice, quinoa, and oats provide fiber and essential nutrients without excessively taxing the kidneys. These grains can help regulate blood sugar and reduce the risk of CKD progression.

- **Low-Potassium Fruits and Vegetables:** Apples, cranberries, and cucumbers are lower in potassium and safe to consume in moderation. These foods support kidney function while keeping potassium levels balanced.

- **Calcium-Rich Foods:** Low-phosphorus dairy alternatives like almond milk or rice milk can provide calcium without overloading the kidneys with phosphorus. Leafy greens like kale and fortified tofu also contribute to calcium intake.

- **Herbs and Spices:** Fresh herbs like parsley, cilantro, and basil, along with spices like turmeric and ginger, can enhance flavor without adding sodium. They also contain antioxidants that support overall health.

- **Water and Hydration:** Staying hydrated is essential, but it's important to manage fluid intake according to your healthcare provider's advice. In general, water is the best choice for hydration. If allowed, herbal teas and small amounts of fruit-infused water can add variety without excess sugar or potassium.

FOODS TO AVOID OR LIMIT

For individuals with CKD, it's crucial to be mindful of foods that can exacerbate the condition. Here's a list of foods to avoid or consume sparingly:

- **High-Sodium Foods:** Processed meats, canned soups, salted snacks, fast food, and frozen dinners are often high in sodium, which can strain the kidneys and elevate blood pressure.

- **High-Potassium Foods:** Bananas, oranges, potatoes, tomatoes, and spinach are rich in potassium, which can be dangerous if not properly managed. Limiting these foods or using specific preparation techniques, like leaching, can help reduce potassium content.

- **High-Phosphorus Foods:** Dairy products, nuts, seeds, beans, and colas are high in phosphorus, which can accumulate in the blood if the kidneys are not functioning well. Phosphorus additives found in processed foods should also be avoided.

- **Red Meat:** While it is a source of high-quality protein, red meat can be hard on the kidneys due to its high phosphorus content and potential to increase inflammation. It's best to consume red meat in moderation and focus on leaner protein sources like fish or poultry.

- **Processed and Convenience Foods:** Many convenience foods contain preservatives and additives that are harmful to kidney health. These often include excess sodium, potassium, and phosphorus, which can exacerbate CKD symptoms.

- **Sugary Foods and Drinks:** High-sugar foods and beverages, including sodas, candy, and baked goods, can contribute to weight gain, diabetes, and high blood pressure, all of which negatively impact kidney health.

- **Alcohol:** Excessive alcohol intake can damage kidneys and worsen existing CKD. If you choose to drink, do so in moderation, following your healthcare provider's guidelines.

PERSONALIZED DIETARY GUIDANCE

Since each individual's experience with CKD is unique, personalized dietary advice is essential. Working with a registered dietitian or nutritionist specialized in kidney health can help you develop a meal plan tailored to your specific needs, preferences, and CKD stage. This customized approach ensures that your diet supports your overall health while effectively managing your kidney condition.

THE ROLE OF EXERCISE IN CKD MANAGEMENT

In addition to dietary adjustments, regular physical activity is crucial in managing CKD. Exercise helps maintain a healthy weight, control blood pressure, and improve overall cardiovascular health—all vital aspects of CKD management.

- **Types of Exercise:** Low-impact activities such as walking, swimming, cycling, and yoga are excellent choices for individuals with CKD. These exercises are gentle on the joints while promoting cardiovascular health.

- **Exercise Frequency:** Aim for at least 30 minutes of moderate exercise most days of the week. However, it's essential to listen to your body and avoid overexertion. If you're new to exercise or have any concerns, consult your healthcare provider before starting a new routine.

- **Strength Training:** Incorporating strength training exercises, such as light weightlifting or resistance band workouts, can help maintain muscle mass and strength, which is especially important for individuals with CKD who may be at risk of muscle loss.

- **Flexibility and Balance:** Activities like stretching and balance exercises can enhance mobility and reduce the risk of falls, which is particularly beneficial for older adults or those with limited mobility due to CKD.

REGULAR MONITORING AND MEDICAL CHECK-UPS

Routine check-ups and lab tests are integral to managing CKD. Regular monitoring allows your healthcare team to assess your kidney function, track the progression of the disease, and make necessary adjustments to your treatment plan.

- **Blood Tests:** These can measure levels of waste products, electrolytes, and other markers of kidney function, such as creatinine and urea.

- **Urine Tests:** Urine analysis can reveal the presence of protein, blood, or other substances that indicate kidney damage.

- **Blood Pressure Monitoring:** Keeping your blood pressure in check is crucial. High blood pressure can accelerate kidney damage, so regular monitoring and appropriate medication are often necessary.

- **Medication Management:** Taking medications as prescribed, especially those for blood pressure, diabetes, and cholesterol, is vital in slowing CKD progression. Always consult your healthcare provider before starting or stopping any medication.

SUPPORT AND RESOURCES

Managing CKD can be challenging, but you don't have to do it alone. Many resources are available to help you navigate your journey with CKD:

- **Support Groups:** Connecting with others who have CKD can provide emotional support and practical advice. Consider joining a local or online support group where you can share experiences and learn from others.

- **Educational Materials:** Books, websites, and webinars can offer valuable information about living with CKD. Reliable sources include the National Kidney Foundation and the American Association of Kidney Patients.

- **Professional Counseling:** If you're feeling overwhelmed, speaking with a mental health professional can help you cope with the emotional aspects of living with a chronic illness.

- **Nutritional Counseling:** Regular consultations with a dietitian specializing in renal nutrition can ensure that your diet continues to meet your evolving needs as CKD progresses.

Chronic Kidney Disease requires careful management, but with the right approach, you can maintain a good quality of life. By understanding CKD, making informed dietary choices, staying active, and working closely with your healthcare team, you can slow the progression of the disease and protect your kidney health. Remember, every small step you take in managing CKD brings you closer to living a healthier, more fulfilling life.

SMOOTHIES

Spinach and Pineapple Smoothie

This smoothie combines the refreshing taste of pineapple with the nutritional benefits of spinach, creating a healthy and balanced drink.

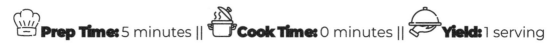 **Prep Time:** 5 minutes || **Cook Time:** 0 minutes || **Yield:** 1 serving

INGREDIENTS

- 1 cup fresh spinach
- 1/2 cup pineapple chunks (fresh or frozen)
- 1/2 cup unsweetened almond milk
- 1/4 cup plain Greek yogurt
- Stevia or monk fruit sweetener to taste (optional)
- Ice cubes

INSTRUCTIONS:

1. Combine spinach, pineapple chunks, almond milk, Greek yogurt, and sweetener (if using) in a blender.

2. Blend until smooth and desired consistency is reached.

3. Add ice cubes and blend again until smooth.

NOTES:

- For a sweeter taste, add a ripe banana to the smoothie.
- You can adjust the thickness by adding more or less liquid.
- For extra protein, add a scoop of plant-based protein powder.

NUTRITIONAL INFO (approximate per serving):

- Calories: 150-200 | Protein: 6-8 g | Fat: 2-4 g | Carbohydrates: 15-20 g | Sodium: 10-20 mg (may vary based on ingredients) | Potassium: 200-300 mg | Phosphorus: 50-70 mg

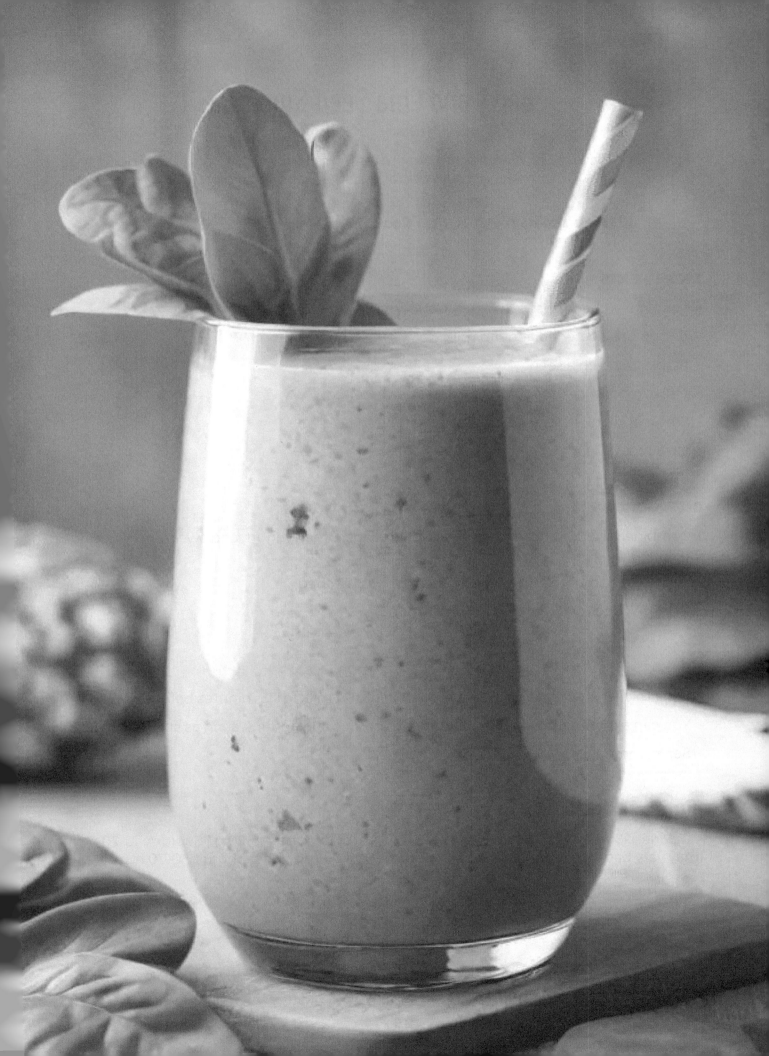

Berry and Chia Seed Smoothie

This recipe focuses on using natural sweetness from berries and minimizing added sugars, making it suitable for a diabetic and renal diet.

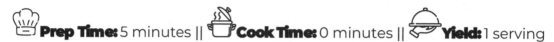 **Prep Time:** 5 minutes || **Cook Time:** 0 minutes || **Yield:** 1 serving

INGREDIENTS

- 1 cup mixed berries (strawberries, raspberries, blueberries)
- 1/2 cup unsweetened almond milk
- 1 tablespoon chia seeds
- 1 tablespoon Greek yogurt (plain and unsweetened)
- Stevia or monk fruit sweetener to taste (optional)
- Ice cubes

INSTRUCTIONS:

1. Combine mixed berries, almond milk, chia seeds, Greek yogurt, and sweetener (if using) in a blender.

2. Blend until smooth and desired consistency is reached.

3. Add ice cubes and blend again until smooth.

NOTES:

- For a thicker smoothie, soak chia seeds in almond milk for 15 minutes before blending.
- You can experiment with different types of berries and add-ins, such as spinach or kale.
- Serve immediately for best flavor.

NUTRITIONAL INFO (approximate per serving):

- Calories: 150-200 | Protein: 6-8 g | Fat: 2-4 g | Carbohydrates: 15-20 g | Sodium: 10-20 mg (may vary based on ingredients) | Potassium: 200-300 mg | Phosphorus: 50-70 mg

Cucumber and Mint Infused Water

This recipe is more of a suggestion than a traditional recipe format, as it involves infusing water with flavor rather than cooking ingredients.

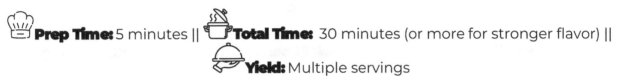

Prep Time: 5 minutes || **Total Time:** 30 minutes (or more for stronger flavor) || **Yield:** Multiple servings

INGREDIENTS

- 1 cucumber, sliced
- A handful of fresh mint leaves
- Filtered water

INSTRUCTIONS:

1. Fill a pitcher with filtered water.
2. Add sliced cucumber and fresh mint leaves to the water.
3. Refrigerate for at least 30 minutes, or longer for a stronger flavor.
4. Serve chilled.

NOTES:

- For additional flavor, add a squeeze of lime or lemon juice.
- You can experiment with different fruits and herbs to create your own infused water variations.
- Infused water is a great way to stay hydrated and add flavor to your water intake.

NUTRITIONAL INFO (approximate per serving):

- Calories: Negligible | Protein: 0 g | Fat: 0 g | Carbohydrates: Negligible | Sodium: 0 mg | Potassium: Low | Phosphorus: Low

Avocado Smoothie

Avocado smoothies can be a healthy option, but it's essential to control portion sizes due to the fat content. This recipe focuses on balancing nutrients while considering the dietary restrictions.

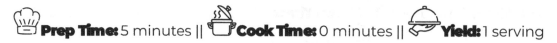 **Prep Time:** 5 minutes || **Cook Time:** 0 minutes || **Yield:** 1 serving

INGREDIENTS

- 1/2 ripe avocado

- 1/2 cup unsweetened almond milk

- 1/4 cup plain Greek yogurt

- 1 tablespoon lemon juice

- Stevia or monk fruit sweetener to taste (optional)

- A handful of spinach or kale (optional)

- Ice cubes

INSTRUCTIONS:

1. Combine avocado, almond milk, Greek yogurt, lemon juice, and sweetener (if using) in a blender.

2. Blend until smooth.

3. Add spinach or kale (if using) and ice cubes. Blend again until desired consistency is reached.

NOTES:

- For a thicker smoothie, use less almond milk or add frozen fruit.

- You can experiment with different flavor combinations by adding a sprinkle of cinnamon or nutmeg.

- Serve immediately for best flavor.

NUTRITIONAL INFO (approximate per serving):

- Calories: 200-250 | Protein: 6-8 g | Fat: 12-15 g | Carbohydrates: 10-15 g | Sodium: 10-20 mg (may vary based on ingredients) | Potassium: 300-400 mg | Phosphorus: 50-70 mg

Protein Smoothie

Traditional protein smoothies often contain high amounts of sugar and added ingredients that may not be suitable for a diabetic and renal diet. This recipe focuses on using natural protein sources and minimizing added sugars.

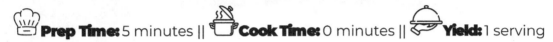 **Prep Time:** 5 minutes || **Cook Time:** 0 minutes || **Yield:** 1 serving

INGREDIENTS

- 1/2 cup Greek yogurt (plain and unsweetened)
- 1 scoop protein powder (unflavored or vanilla)
- 1/2 cup unsweetened almond milk
- 1/2 banana (frozen for a thicker consistency)
- A handful of spinach or kale (optional)
- Stevia or monk fruit sweetener to taste (optional)
- Ice cubes

INSTRUCTIONS:

1. Combine Greek yogurt, protein powder, almond milk, banana, spinach or kale (if using), and sweetener (if using) in a blender.

2. Blend until smooth and desired consistency is reached.

3. Add ice cubes and blend again until smooth.

NOTES:

- For additional protein, you can add a spoonful of chia seeds or flaxseed meal.
- Experiment with different fruits and greens to create your own flavor combinations.
- You can adjust the thickness of the smoothie by adding more or less liquid.

NUTRITIONAL INFO (approximate per serving):

- Calories: 150-200 | Protein: 15-20 g | Fat: 2-4 g | Carbohydrates: 10-15 g | Sodium: 10-20 mg (may vary based on ingredients) | Potassium: 200-300 mg | Phosphorus: 50-70 mg

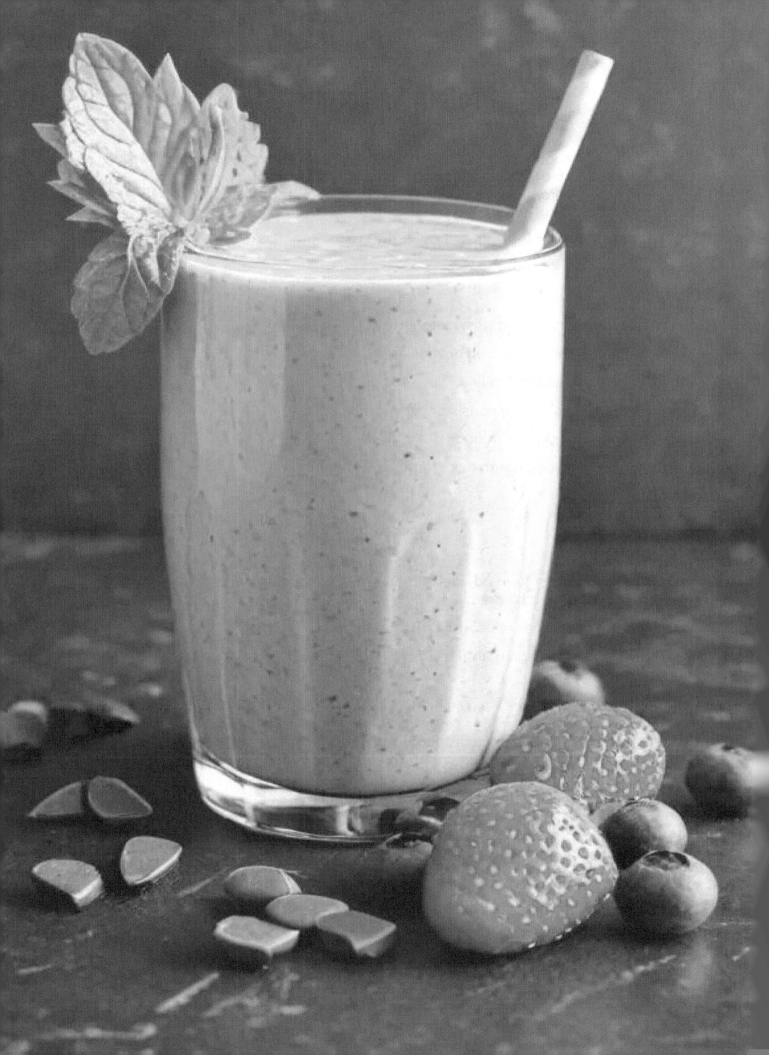

Green Smoothie

Traditional green smoothies often include ingredients that are not suitable for a diabetic and renal diet, such as excessive sugar and high-sodium ingredients. This recipe offers a modified version that is lower in sugar and sodium.

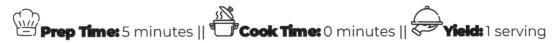 **Prep Time:** 5 minutes || **Cook Time:** 0 minutes || **Yield:** 1 serving

INGREDIENTS

- 1 cup spinach or kale
- 1/2 cup unsweetened almond milk
- 1/2 banana (frozen for a thicker consistency)
- 1 tablespoon Greek yogurt (plain and unsweetened)
- Stevia or monk fruit sweetener to taste (optional)
- A handful of ice cubes

INSTRUCTIONS:

1. Combine spinach or kale, almond milk, banana, Greek yogurt, and sweetener (if using) in a blender.

2. Blend until smooth and desired consistency is reached.

3. Add ice cubes and blend again until smooth.

NOTES:

- For added flavor, you can include a squeeze of lemon or lime juice.
- You can experiment with different greens, such as romaine lettuce or collard greens.
- For a thicker smoothie, add more frozen banana or spinach.

NUTRITIONAL INFO (approximate per serving):

- Calories: 150-200 | Protein: 6-8 g | Fat: 2-4 g | Carbohydrates: 15-20 g | Sodium: 10-20 mg (may vary based on ingredients) | Potassium: 200-300 mg | Phosphorus: 50-70 mg

SNACKS & DESSERTS

Rice Cakes or Whole-Grain Crackers with Low-Sodium Toppings

This recipe is less a recipe and more a suggestion for a quick and healthy snack option.

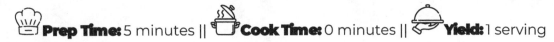 **Prep Time:** 5 minutes || **Cook Time:** 0 minutes || **Yield:** 1 serving

INGREDIENTS

- 1 rice cake or whole-grain cracker
- 1 tablespoon low-sodium hummus or mashed avocado
- Optional toppings: sliced cucumber, cherry tomatoes, red onion

INSTRUCTIONS:

1. Spread hummus or mashed avocado on the rice cake or whole-grain cracker.

2. Add desired toppings, such as sliced cucumber, cherry tomatoes, or red onion.

NOTES:

- Choose rice cakes or whole-grain crackers that are low in sodium.
- For added protein, top with a sprinkle of chia seeds or hemp hearts.
- Experiment with different toppings to create your own flavor combinations.

NUTRITIONAL INFO (approximate per serving):

- Calories: 100-150 | Protein: 2-4 g | Fat: 5-8 g | Carbohydrates: 15-20 g | Sodium: 100-150 mg (may vary based on ingredients) | Potassium: 200-300 mg | Phosphorus: 100-150 mg

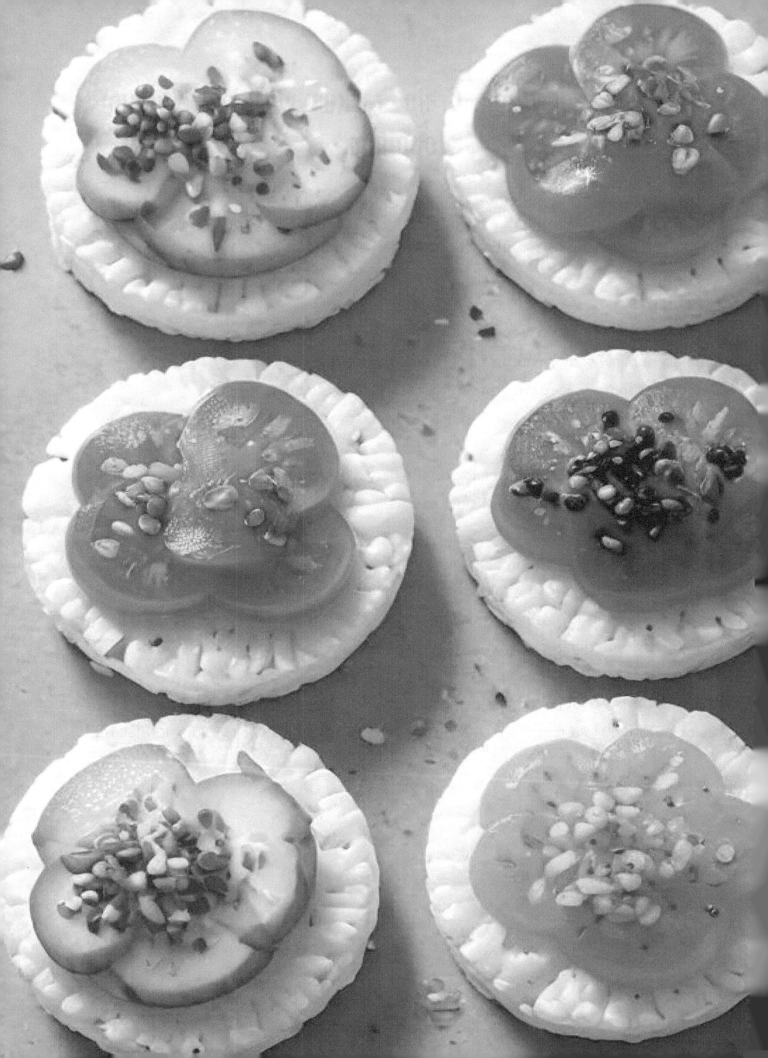

Fresh Fruit Sorbet

Traditional sorbet recipes often rely on high amounts of sugar. This recipe offers a modified version that is lower in sugar and suitable for a diabetic and renal diet.

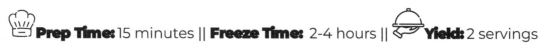 **Prep Time:** 15 minutes || **Freeze Time:** 2-4 hours || **Yield:** 2 servings

INGREDIENTS

- 2 cups mixed berries (strawberries, raspberries, blueberries)
- 1/2 cup unsweetened Greek yogurt
- 1 tablespoon lemon juice
- Stevia or monk fruit sweetener to taste (optional)

INSTRUCTIONS:

1. In a food processor or blender, combine mixed berries, Greek yogurt, lemon juice, and sweetener (if using).

2. Blend until smooth.

3. Pour the mixture into a freezer-safe container and freeze for 2-4 hours, or until firm.

4. Stir the sorbet every 30 minutes to prevent large ice crystals from forming.

NOTES:

- For a creamier texture, add a splash of coconut milk or almond milk.
- Experiment with different fruit combinations, such as mango, pineapple, or peach.
- Serve immediately for a soft sorbet or let freeze for a longer period for a harder texture.

NUTRITIONAL INFO (approximate per serving):

- Calories: 100-150 | Protein: 3-5 g | Fat: 2-4 g | Carbohydrates: 15-20 g | Sodium: 10-20 mg (may vary based on ingredients) | Potassium: 200-300 mg | Phosphorus: 50-70 mg

Baked Apples

Traditional baked apples often involve excessive sugar and butter. This recipe offers a modified version that is lower in sugar and fat.

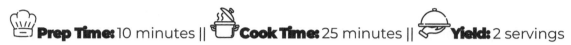 **Prep Time:** 10 minutes || **Cook Time:** 25 minutes || **Yield:** 2 servings

INGREDIENTS

- 2 large apples (Granny Smith or Honeycrisp)

- 1 tablespoon sugar-free apple jelly or preserves (optional)

- 1/4 teaspoon ground cinnamon

- Pinch of nutmeg

- Optional toppings: a dollop of plain Greek yogurt or a sprinkle of nuts

INSTRUCTIONS:

1. Preheat oven to 375°F (190°C).

2. Core apples without cutting all the way through the bottom.

3. Fill the apple centers with sugar-free apple jelly or preserves, if using.

4. Sprinkle cinnamon and nutmeg over the apple filling.

5. Place apples in a baking dish and add a small amount of water to the bottom of the dish to prevent drying.

6. Bake for 25-30 minutes, or until apples are tender.

7. Serve warm with optional toppings.

NOTES:

- For additional sweetness, you can sprinkle a small amount of stevia or monk fruit sweetener over the apple filling.

- You can add a sprinkle of ground cloves or cardamom for extra flavor.

- Serve with a scoop of sugar-free vanilla ice cream for a dessert option.

NUTRITIONAL INFO (approximate per serving):

- Calories: 100-150 | Protein: 1-2 g | Fat: 0-1 g | Carbohydrates: 20-25 g | Sodium: 10-20 mg (may vary based on ingredients) | Potassium: 200-300 mg | Phosphorus: 50-70 mg

Fruit Crumble

Traditional fruit crumbles often contain high amounts of sugar and butter, which are not suitable for a diabetic and renal diet. This recipe offers a modified version with reduced sugar and fat content.

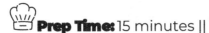 **Prep Time:** 15 minutes || 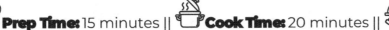 **Cook Time:** 20 minutes || 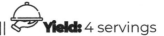 **Yield:** 4 servings

INGREDIENTS

For the Fruit Filling:

- 4 cups mixed berries (blueberries, raspberries, blackberries)

- 1 tablespoon cornstarch

- 1 tablespoon lemon juice

- Sweetener to taste (optional, such as stevia or monk fruit)

For the Crumble Topping:

- 1/2 cup whole-wheat flour

- 1/4 cup rolled oats

- 1/4 cup almond flour

- 1 tablespoon ground cinnamon

- Pinch of nutmeg

- 1 tablespoon olive oil

INSTRUCTIONS:

1. Preheat oven to 375°F (190°C).

2. In a large bowl, combine mixed berries, cornstarch, lemon juice, and sweetener (if using).

3. In a separate bowl, combine crumble topping ingredients.

4. Pour fruit filling into a baking dish. Sprinkle crumble topping evenly over the fruit.

5. Bake for 20-25 minutes, or until fruit is bubbling and crumble topping is golden brown.

NOTES:

- Serve warm with a scoop of low-fat Greek yogurt or a dollop of sugar-free whipped cream (optional).

- You can use other fruits, such as apples, pears, or peaches, as the base for your crumble.

NUTRITIONAL INFO (approximate per serving):

- Calories: 150-200 | Protein: 2-4 g | Fat: 5-8 g | Carbohydrates: 25-30 g | Sodium: 100-150 mg (may vary based on ingredients) | Potassium: 200-300 mg | Phosphorus: 100-150 mg

Rice Pudding

Traditional rice pudding often includes ingredients that are not suitable for a diabetic and renal diet, such as excessive sugar and whole milk. This recipe offers a modified version that is lower in sugar and fat.

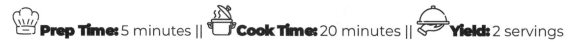 **Prep Time:** 5 minutes || **Cook Time:** 20 minutes || **Yield:** 2 servings

INGREDIENTS

- 1/2 cup white rice
- 1 cup unsweetened almond milk
- 1/4 teaspoon cinnamon
- Pinch of salt
- Optional: Stevia or monk fruit sweetener to taste
- Optional: A sprinkle of ground nutmeg for flavor

INSTRUCTIONS:

1. In a medium saucepan, combine rice, almond milk, cinnamon, and salt.

2. Bring to a boil, then reduce heat to low and simmer for 15-20 minutes, or until rice is tender and liquid is absorbed.

3. Stir occasionally to prevent sticking.

4. If desired, sweeten with a small amount of stevia or monk fruit sweetener.

5. Let cool slightly before serving.

NOTES:

- For a thicker pudding, cook for a few extra minutes.
- You can add a sprinkle of ground nutmeg or vanilla extract for additional flavor.
- Serve chilled or warm, depending on your preference.

NUTRITIONAL INFO (approximate per serving):

- Calories: 150-200 | Protein: 3-5 g | Fat: 2-4 g | Carbohydrates: 30-35 g | Sodium: 100-150 mg (may vary based on ingredients) | Potassium: 200-300 mg | Phosphorus: 100-150 mg

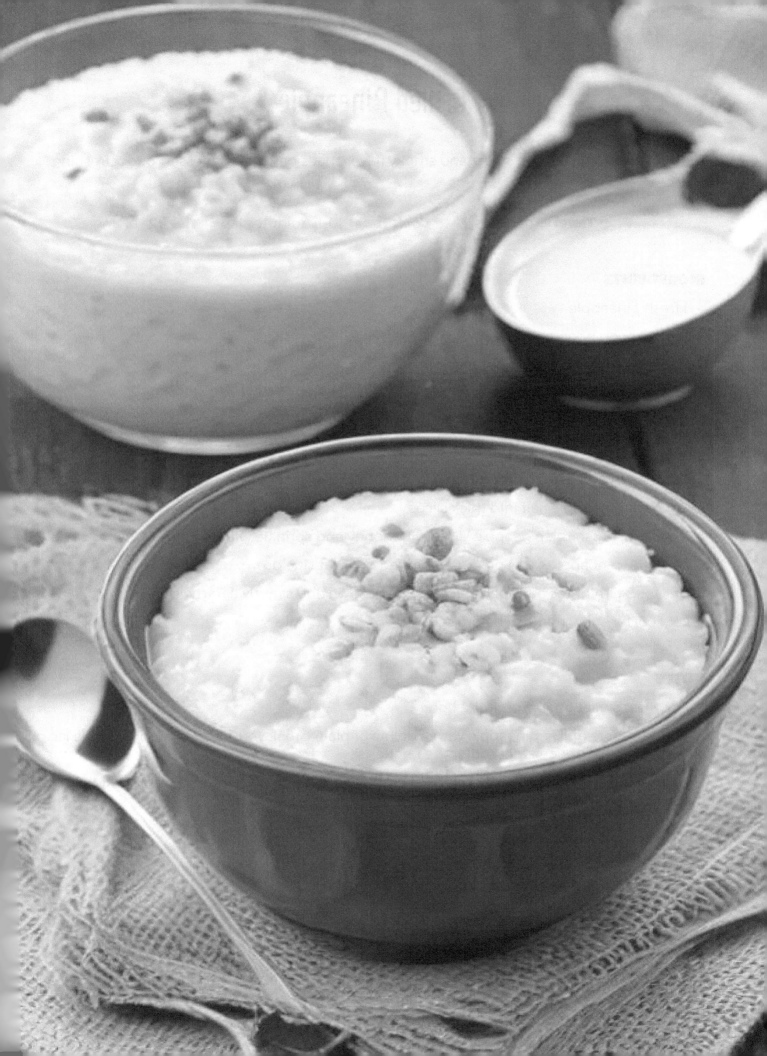

Grilled Pineapple

Grilled pineapple offers a sweet and smoky flavor that's perfect as a dessert or a refreshing side dish.

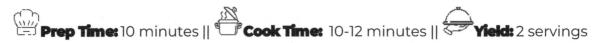 **Prep Time:** 10 minutes || **Cook Time:** 10-12 minutes || **Yield:** 2 servings

INGREDIENTS

- 1 fresh pineapple

- 1 tablespoon honey (optional)

- 1/2 teaspoon ground cinnamon

INSTRUCTIONS

1. Preheat your grill to medium-high heat.

2. Cut the pineapple in half lengthwise and remove the hard core.

3. Cut each pineapple half into thick slices.

4. If desired, brush the pineapple slices with honey and sprinkle with cinnamon.

5. Place the pineapple slices on the preheated grill, cut side down.

6. Grill for 5-6 minutes per side, or until golden brown and slightly caramelized.

7. Let cool for a few minutes before serving.

NOTES

- For a less sweet option, omit the honey.

- You can serve grilled pineapple with a dollop of plain Greek yogurt or a scoop of vanilla ice cream (for those not on strict sodium restrictions).

- Be mindful of the potassium content in pineapple, especially for individuals with kidney disease.

NUTRITIONAL INFO (per serving):

- Calories: 70 | Protein: 1g | Fat: 0g | Carbohydrates: 17g | Sodium: 0mg | Potassium: 200mg | Phosphorus: 10mg

Vegetable Sticks with Hummus

This simple and satisfying snack is packed with vitamins, minerals, and fiber. Hummus provides protein and healthy fats, while the vegetables offer essential nutrients.

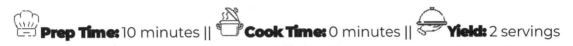 **Prep Time:** 10 minutes || **Cook Time:** 0 minutes || **Yield:** 2 servings

INGREDIENTS

- 1 cup carrots, sliced
- 1 cup celery sticks
- 1 cup cucumber sticks
- 1/2 cup red bell pepper strips
- 1/2 cup low-sodium hummus

INSTRUCTIONS

1. Prepare the vegetables by washing, peeling, and cutting them into sticks.
2. Serve the vegetable sticks with hummus in a serving bowl or on individual plates.

NOTES

- Choose fresh, crisp vegetables for optimal taste and texture.
- For added flavor, sprinkle the vegetables with a pinch of garlic powder or onion powder.
- You can vary the vegetables based on your preferences and what's available.

VARIATIONS

- Add a sprinkle of paprika or cumin to the hummus for extra flavor.
- Serve with whole-grain pita bread for a more substantial snack.
- For a lower-calorie option, use a reduced-fat hummus.

NUTRITIONAL INFO (per serving):

- Calories: 150 | Protein: 5g | Fat: 6g | Carbohydrates: 15g | Sodium: 100mg | Potassium: 250mg | Phosphorus: 80mg

Clementines

Clementines are a simple yet nutritious snack, rich in vitamin C and other essential nutrients. They are naturally low in sodium and potassium, making them a suitable choice for people on a renal diet.

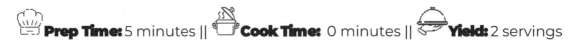 **Prep Time:** 5 minutes || **Cook Time:** 0 minutes || **Yield:** 2 servings

INGREDIENTS

- 4 clementines

INSTRUCTIONS

1. Wash the clementines thoroughly under cold water.

2. Peel the clementines and separate into segments.

3. Serve immediately.

NOTES

- Clementines are a versatile fruit that can be enjoyed on their own or added to salads, yogurt, or oatmeal.

- For added flavor, sprinkle a little cinnamon or nutmeg on top.

- To reduce mess, peel clementines over a bowl to catch any juice.

NUTRITIONAL INFO (per serving):

- Calories: 50 | Protein: 1g | Fat: 0g | Carbohydrates: 12g | Sodium: 0mg | Potassium: 150mg | Phosphorus: 10mg

Fruit Salsa and Sweet Chips

This fresh and vibrant combination offers a sweet and satisfying snack or dessert. The fruit salsa is packed with vitamins and antioxidants, while the sweet potato chips provide a healthy crunch.

Fruit Salsa

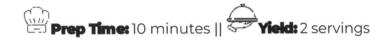 **Prep Time:** 10 minutes || **Yield:** 2 servings

INGREDIENTS

- 1 cup diced mango
- 1 cup diced pineapple
- 1/2 cup diced strawberries
- 1 tablespoon lime juice
- 1 teaspoon orange zest (optional)

INSTRUCTIONS

1. In a medium bowl, combine mango, pineapple, and strawberries.

2. Stir in lime juice and orange zest (if using).

3. Serve immediately or chill for later.

Sweet Potato Chips

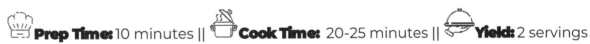 **Prep Time:** 10 minutes || **Cook Time:** 20-25 minutes || **Yield:** 2 servings

INGREDIENTS

- 1 large sweet potato
- 1 tablespoon olive oil
- 1/4 teaspoon cinnamon
- Pinch of salt

INSTRUCTIONS

1. Preheat oven to 400°F (200°C).

2. Peel and thinly slice the sweet potato.

3. Toss the sweet potato slices with olive oil, cinnamon, and salt.

4. Spread the slices in a single layer on a baking sheet lined with parchment paper.

5. Bake for 20-25 minutes, or until crispy.

6. Let cool completely before serving.

Serving Suggestions:

Serve the fruit salsa and sweet potato chips together for a refreshing and satisfying snack.

NOTES

- For the sweet potato chips, you can experiment with different seasonings, such as garlic powder, paprika, or chili powder.

- Be mindful of the potassium content in fruits, especially for individuals with kidney disease.

- Store leftover fruit salsa in the refrigerator for up to 2 days.

NUTRITIONAL INFO (approximate, per serving):

- **Fruit Salsa:** Calories: 100 | Protein: 1g | Fat: 1g | Carbohydrates: 25g | Sodium: 5mg | Potassium: 300mg | Phosphorus: 20mg

- **Sweet Potato Chips:** Calories: 150 | Protein: 2g | Fat: 7g | Carbohydrates: 20g | Sodium: 50mg | Potassium: 350mg | Phosphorus: 50mg

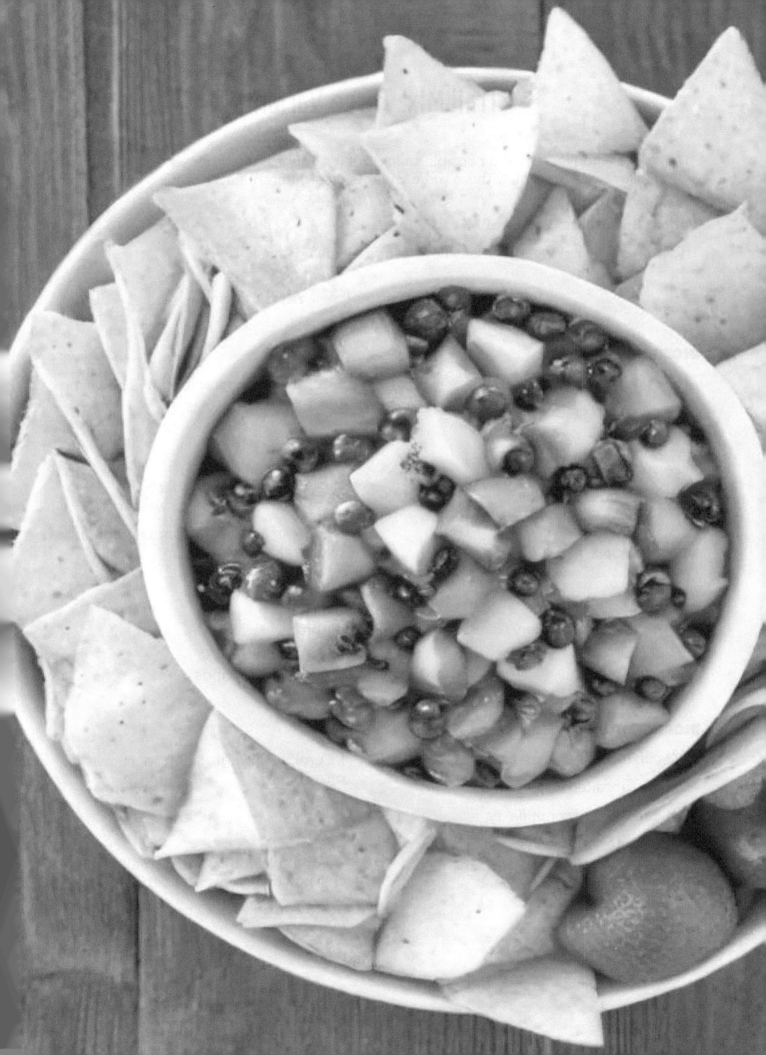

Trail Mix: Three Variants

Trail mix is a convenient and portable snack, but it's important to choose ingredients wisely when following a renal diet. These three variants offer different flavor profiles while adhering to dietary restrictions.

Variant 1: Sweet and Salty Trail Mix

This mix combines sweet and salty flavors for a satisfying snack.

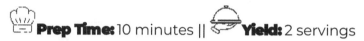 **Prep Time:** 10 minutes || **Yield:** 2 servings

INGREDIENTS

- 1/2 cup unsalted almonds
- 1/4 cup dried cranberries
- 1/4 cup sunflower seeds
- 1/4 cup dried apricots
- 1/4 cup pumpkin seeds

INSTRUCTIONS

1. Combine all ingredients in a bowl and mix well.

NOTES

- Choose dried fruits that are unsweetened or lightly sweetened.
- Store in an airtight container for up to two weeks.

Variant 2: Savory Trail Mix

This mix focuses on savory flavors with a crunchy texture.

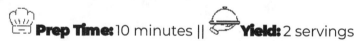 **Prep Time:** 10 minutes || **Yield:** 2 servings

INGREDIENTS

- 1/2 cup roasted chickpeas
- 1/4 cup unsalted cashews
- 1/4 cup dried coconut flakes
- 1/4 cup pumpkin seeds
- 1/4 cup dried rosemary

INSTRUCTIONS

1. Combine all ingredients in a bowl and mix well.

NOTES

- For a spicier mix, add a small amount of chili powder or cayenne pepper.
- Store in an airtight container for up to two weeks.

Variant 3: Energy Boost Trail Mix

This mix combines nuts, seeds, and dried fruit for a sustained energy boost.

Prep Time: 10 minutes || **Yield:** 2 servings

INGREDIENTS

- 1/2 cup walnuts
- 1/4 cup chia seeds
- 1/4 cup raisins
- 1/4 cup dried figs
- 1/4 cup flax seeds

INSTRUCTIONS

1. Combine all ingredients in a bowl and mix well.

NOTES

- Chia and flax seeds are rich in omega-3 fatty acids, which are beneficial for heart health.
- Store in an airtight container in the refrigerator for freshness.

GENERAL NOTES FOR ALL VARIANTS:

- Monitor potassium intake, especially for dried fruits.
- Adjust quantities based on personal preference.
- Store trail mix in an airtight container to maintain freshness.

NUTRITIONAL INFORMATION (approximate, per serving):

- Calories: 200-300 | Protein: 5-8g | Fat: 12-15g | Carbohydrates: 20-25g | Sodium: Varies based on ingredients | Potassium: Varies based on ingredients | Phosphorus: Varies based on ingredients

Cranberry Orange Muffins

These muffins offer a burst of flavor with the combination of tart cranberries and zesty orange. They are a healthier alternative to traditional muffins, with a focus on whole grains and reduced sugar.

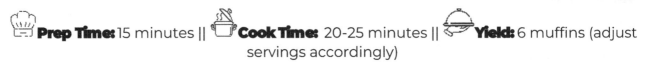 **Prep Time:** 15 minutes || **Cook Time:** 20-25 minutes || **Yield:** 6 muffins (adjust servings accordingly)

INGREDIENTS

- 1 cup whole wheat flour
- 1/2 teaspoon baking powder
- 1/4 teaspoon baking soda
- 1/4 teaspoon ground cinnamon
- 1/4 teaspoon salt
- 1/4 cup unsweetened applesauce
- 1/4 cup maple syrup (or sugar substitute)
- 1 egg white
- 1/4 cup plain Greek yogurt
- 1/4 cup dried cranberries
- 1 tablespoon orange zest

INSTRUCTIONS

1. Preheat oven to 375°F (190°C). Line a muffin tin with paper liners.

2. In a large bowl, whisk together whole wheat flour, baking powder, baking soda, cinnamon, and salt.

3. In a separate bowl, combine applesauce, maple syrup, egg white, and Greek yogurt.

4. Gradually add wet ingredients to dry ingredients, mixing until just combined. Stir in dried cranberries and orange zest.

5. Divide batter evenly among muffin cups.

6. Bake for 20-25 minutes, or until a toothpick inserted into the center comes out clean.

7. Let cool in muffin tin for a few minutes before transferring to a wire rack to cool completely.

NOTES

- For a moister muffin, add an extra tablespoon of applesauce.

- Fresh cranberries can be used instead of dried, but they will require additional cooking time.

- You can add a tablespoon of orange juice to the batter for extra flavor.

NUTRITIONAL INFO (per muffin, approximate):

- Calories: 120 | Protein: 3g | Fat: 3g | Carbohydrates: 20g | Sodium: 50mg | Potassium: 150mg | Phosphorus: 50mg

Three-Grain Raspberry Muffins

These muffins offer a nutritious and flavorful treat, combining the benefits of three different grains for a complex carbohydrate base. The addition of raspberries provides a burst of antioxidants.

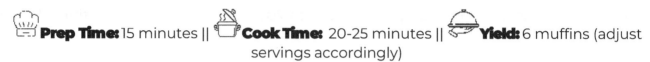

Prep Time: 15 minutes || **Cook Time:** 20-25 minutes || **Yield:** 6 muffins (adjust servings accordingly)

INGREDIENTS

- 1/2 cup whole wheat flour
- 1/2 cup oat flour
- 1/4 cup cornmeal
- 1/2 teaspoon baking powder
- 1/4 teaspoon baking soda
- 1/4 teaspoon ground cinnamon
- 1/4 teaspoon salt
- 1/4 cup unsweetened applesauce
- 1/4 cup maple syrup (or sugar substitute)
- 1 egg white
- 1/4 cup plain Greek yogurt
- 1/2 cup fresh or frozen raspberries

INSTRUCTIONS

1. Preheat oven to 375°F (190°C). Line a muffin tin with paper liners.

2. In a large bowl, whisk together whole wheat flour, oat flour, cornmeal, baking powder, baking soda, cinnamon, and salt.

3. In a separate bowl, combine applesauce, maple syrup, egg white, and Greek yogurt.

4. Gradually add wet ingredients to dry ingredients, mixing until just combined. Gently fold in raspberries.

5. Divide batter evenly among muffin cups.

6. Bake for 20-25 minutes, or until a toothpick inserted into the center comes out clean.

7. Let cool in muffin tin for a few minutes before transferring to a wire rack to cool completely.

NOTES

- You can substitute fresh raspberries with frozen ones, but the baking time might need to be adjusted slightly.

- For a nuttier flavor, add a handful of chopped almonds or walnuts.

NUTRITIONAL INFO (per muffin, approximate):

- Calories: 120 | Protein: 3g | Fat: 3g | Carbohydrates: 20g | Sodium: 50mg | Potassium: 150mg | Phosphorus: 50mg

PASTA & GRAINS

Brown Rice Pilaf with Chicken and Stir-Fried Vegetables

This dish offers a complete and balanced meal, packed with protein, carbohydrates, and vegetables.

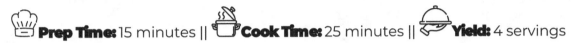 **Prep Time:** 15 minutes || **Cook Time:** 25 minutes || **Yield:** 4 servings

INGREDIENTS

- 1 cup brown rice

- 2 cups chicken broth

- 1/2 onion, chopped

- 1 carrot, diced

- 1 green bell pepper, sliced

- 2 cloves garlic, minced

- 1/2 lb boneless, skinless chicken breast, sliced

- 1/4 cup soy sauce (low-sodium)

- 1 tablespoon cornstarch

- 1 tablespoon water

- Salt and pepper to taste

INSTRUCTIONS:

1. Rinse brown rice and combine with chicken broth in a medium saucepan. Bring to a boil, then reduce heat, cover, and simmer for 20 minutes, or until liquid is absorbed.

2. While rice cooks, heat a large skillet over medium-high heat with a drizzle of olive oil. Add chicken and cook until browned. Remove from skillet and set aside.

3. In the same skillet, sauté onion, carrot, and green bell pepper until softened. Add garlic and cook for 30 seconds more.

4. Stir in soy sauce. In a small bowl, whisk together cornstarch and water; add to skillet and cook until sauce thickens. Return chicken to skillet and coat in sauce.

6. Combine cooked rice with chicken and vegetables. Season with salt and pepper.

NOTES:

- For a vegetarian option, substitute chicken with tofu or chickpeas.

- You can add other vegetables, such as broccoli or snow peas, to the stir-fry.

NUTRITIONAL INFO (approximate per serving):

- Calories: 350-400 | Protein: 25-30 g | Fat: 10-12 g | Carbohydrates: 40-45 g | Sodium: 100-150 mg (may vary based on ingredients) | Potassium: 300-400 mg | Phosphorus: 150-200 mg

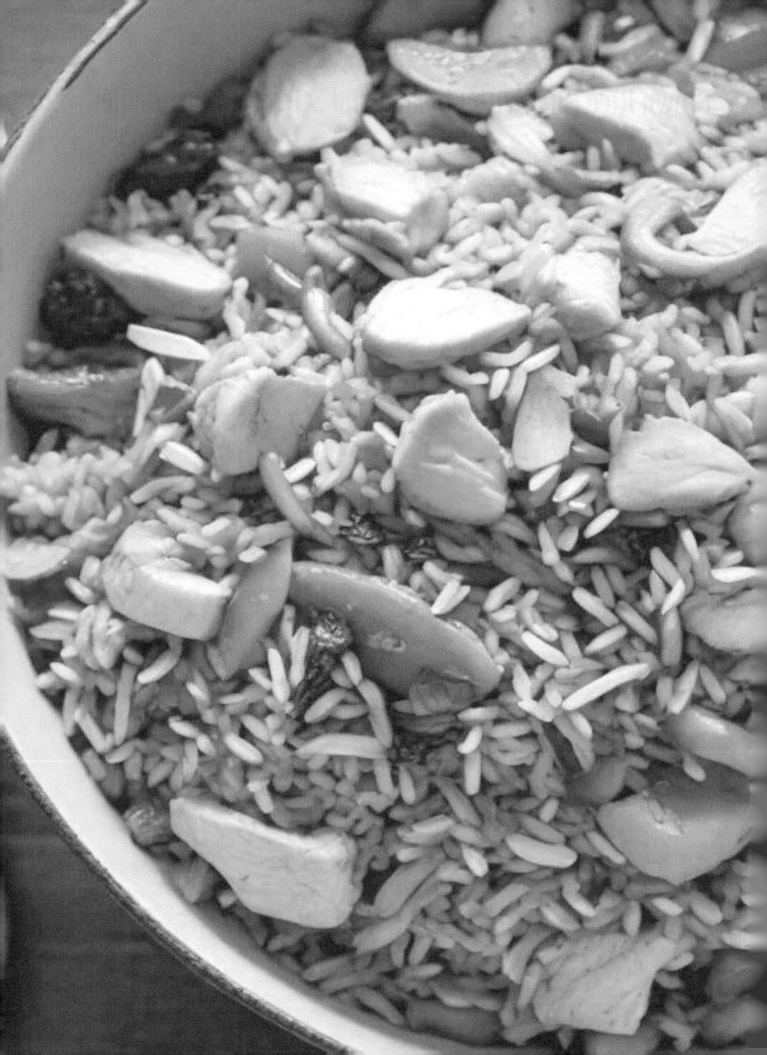

Quinoa Salad with Grilled Salmon and Avocado

This refreshing and satisfying salad is packed with protein and healthy fats.

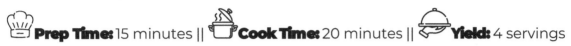 **Prep Time:** 15 minutes || **Cook Time:** 20 minutes || **Yield:** 4 servings

INGREDIENTS

- 1 cup quinoa
- 2 cups vegetable broth
- 4 oz salmon fillet
- 1/2 avocado, diced
- 1/4 cup red onion, finely chopped

- 1/4 cup chopped fresh dill
- 2 tablespoons olive oil
- 1 tablespoon lemon juice
- Salt and pepper to taste

INSTRUCTIONS:

1. Rinse quinoa under cold water.

2. In a medium saucepan, combine quinoa and vegetable broth. Bring to a boil, then reduce heat, cover, and simmer for 15 minutes, or until liquid is absorbed.

3. Fluff quinoa with a fork and let cool completely.

4. Grill salmon until cooked through and flaky. Let cool and flake into chunks.

5. In a large bowl, combine cooked quinoa, diced avocado, red onion, and fresh dill.

6. In a small bowl, whisk together olive oil, lemon juice, salt, and pepper.

7. Pour dressing over the quinoa mixture and toss to coat.

8. Gently stir in grilled salmon.

NOTES:

- For a creamier salad, add a dollop of Greek yogurt or avocado.
- You can add other vegetables, such as cucumber or cherry tomatoes, to the salad.
- Serve chilled for a refreshing summer meal.

NUTRITIONAL INFO (approximate per serving):

- Calories: 300-350 | Protein: 25-30 g | Fat: 10-12 g | Carbohydrates: 30-35 g | Sodium: 100-150 mg (may vary based on ingredients) | Potassium: 300-400 mg | Phosphorus: 150-200 mg

Whole-Wheat Penne with Roasted Red Pepper Pesto

This vibrant pasta dish is a flavorful and healthy option.

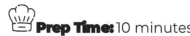**Prep Time:** 10 minutes || 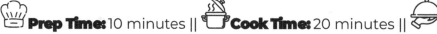**Cook Time:** 20 minutes || 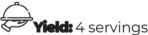**Yield:** 4 servings

INGREDIENTS

- 8 oz whole-wheat penne pasta
- 1 large red bell pepper, roasted and peeled
- 1/2 cup packed fresh basil leaves
- 1/4 cup pine nuts, toasted
- 1/4 cup grated Parmesan cheese (low-sodium)
- 2 cloves garlic
- 1/4 cup olive oil
- Salt and pepper to taste

INSTRUCTIONS:

1. Cook pasta. Drain and reserve 1/4 cup pasta water.

2. While pasta cooks, make the pesto: In a food processor, combine roasted red pepper, basil, pine nuts, Parmesan cheese, garlic, and olive oil. Pulse until smooth. Season with salt and pepper.

3. Combine cooked pasta with pesto in a large bowl. Add reserved pasta water if needed to loosen the sauce.

4. Toss to coat evenly. Serve immediately.

NOTES:

- For a creamier sauce, add a dollop of Greek yogurt or ricotta cheese.
- You can adjust the spice level by adding red pepper flakes to the pesto.
- Serve with grilled chicken or salmon for a more substantial meal.

NUTRITIONAL INFO (approximate per serving):

- Calories: 400-450 | Protein: 15-20 g | Fat: 15-20 g | Carbohydrates: 50-60 g | Sodium: 100-150 mg (may vary based on ingredients) | Potassium: 300-400 mg | Phosphorus: 150-200 mg

Freekeh Pilaf with Chickpeas and Spinach

This hearty and nutritious dish is packed with protein and fiber.

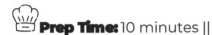 **Prep Time:** 10 minutes || 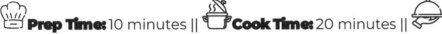 **Cook Time:** 20 minutes || 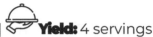 **Yield:** 4 servings

INGREDIENTS

- 1 cup freekeh
- 1 can (15 ounces) chickpeas, drained and rinsed
- 1 onion, chopped
- 2 cloves garlic, minced
- 1 cup vegetable broth

- 1/2 cup fresh spinach, chopped
- 1/4 cup dried cranberries
- 1 tablespoon lemon juice
- 1/2 teaspoon ground cumin
- Salt and pepper to taste

INSTRUCTIONS:

1. Rinse freekeh under cold water.

2. In a medium saucepan, combine freekeh and vegetable broth. Bring to a boil, then reduce heat, cover, and simmer for about 20 minutes, or until freekeh is tender.

3. While freekeh cooks, heat a large skillet over medium heat with a drizzle of olive oil. Sauté onion and garlic until softened.

4. Add chickpeas to the skillet and cook for a few minutes.

5. Combine cooked freekeh, chickpea mixture, spinach, dried cranberries, lemon juice, cumin, salt, and pepper in a large bowl.

6. Toss to combine and serve warm.

NOTES:

- For extra flavor, add toasted pine nuts or slivered almonds.
- You can substitute dried cranberries with other dried fruits, such as apricots or raisins.
- Serve with a side salad or grilled chicken for a complete meal.

NUTRITIONAL INFO (approximate per serving):

- Calories: 300-350 | Protein: 15-20 g | Fat: 5-8 g | Carbohydrates: 40-45 g | Sodium: 100-150 mg (may vary based on ingredients) | Potassium: 300-400 mg | Phosphorus: 150-200 mg

Farro Salad with Grilled Shrimp

This light and refreshing salad is packed with protein and fiber.

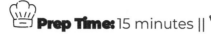**Prep Time:** 15 minutes || 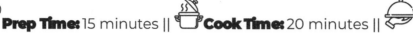**Cook Time:** 20 minutes || 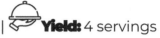**Yield:** 4 servings

INGREDIENTS

- 1 cup farro
- 2 cups vegetable broth
- 1 lb large shrimp, peeled and deveined
- 1/2 cup cherry tomatoes, halved
- 1/4 cup red onion, finely chopped

- 1/4 cup chopped fresh mint
- 2 tablespoons olive oil
- 1 tablespoon lemon juice
- 1/4 teaspoon garlic powder
- Salt and pepper to taste

INSTRUCTIONS:

1. Cook farro, using vegetable broth instead of water. Drain and let cool completely.

2. Grill shrimp until cooked through and pink, about 2-3 minutes per side. Let cool and chop into bite-sized pieces.

3. In a large bowl, combine cooked farro, cherry tomatoes, red onion, and mint.

4. In a small bowl, whisk together olive oil, lemon juice, garlic powder, salt, and pepper.

5. Pour dressing over the farro mixture and toss to coat.

6. Gently stir in grilled shrimp.

NOTES:

- For a creamier salad, add a dollop of Greek yogurt or avocado.
- You can add other vegetables, such as cucumber or bell pepper, to the salad.
- Serve chilled or at room temperature.

NUTRITIONAL INFO (approximate per serving):

- Calories: 300-350 | Protein: 25-30 g | Fat: 10-12 g | Carbohydrates: 35-40 g | Sodium: 100-150 mg (may vary based on ingredients) | Potassium: 300-400 mg | Phosphorus: 150-200 mg

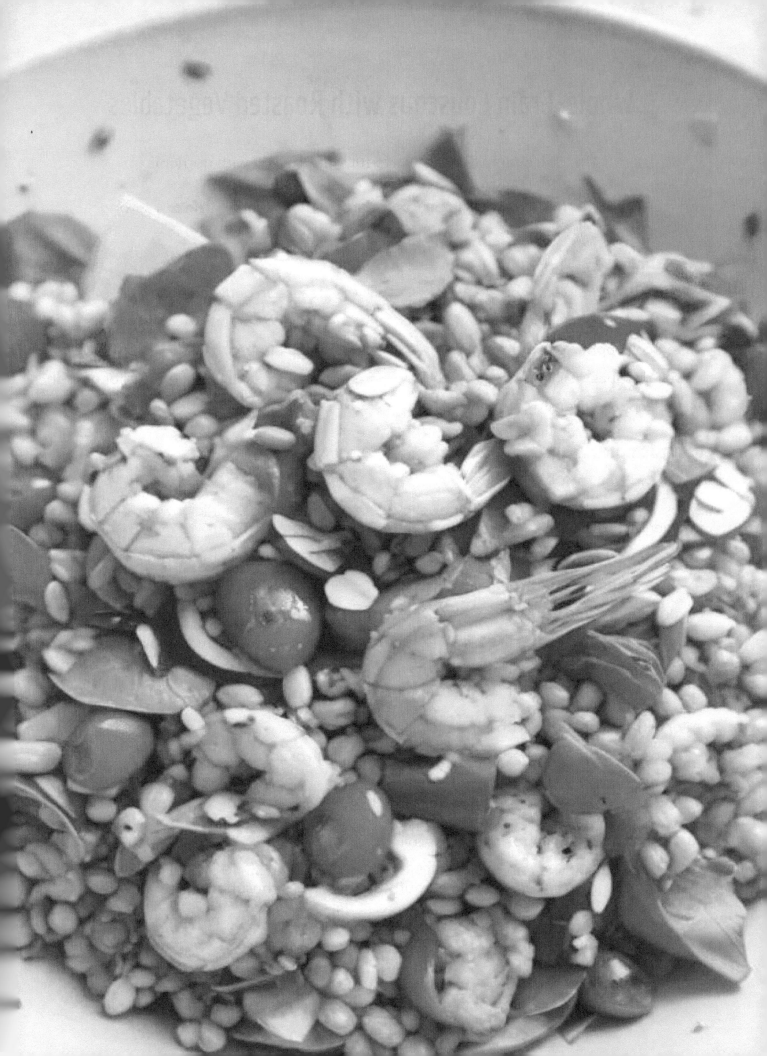

Whole-Grain Couscous with Roasted Vegetables

This dish offers a light and flavorful meal, packed with nutrients.

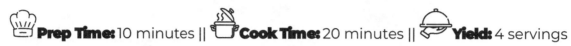 **Prep Time:** 10 minutes || **Cook Time:** 20 minutes || **Yield:** 4 servings

INGREDIENTS

- 1 cup whole-grain couscous
- 1 large sweet potato, cubed
- 1 red bell pepper, cut into chunks
- 1 yellow squash, sliced
- 1 tablespoon olive oil

- 1/2 teaspoon garlic powder
- 1/4 teaspoon onion powder
- Salt and pepper to taste
- Fresh herbs (like basil or mint), for garnish (optional)

INSTRUCTIONS:

1. Preheat oven to 400°F (200°C).

2. Toss sweet potato, bell pepper, and yellow squash with olive oil, garlic powder, onion powder, salt, and pepper on a baking sheet.

3. Roast for 20 minutes, or until vegetables are tender and slightly caramelized.

4. While vegetables roast, prepare couscous.

5. Combine roasted vegetables with cooked couscous in a large bowl.

6. Garnish with fresh herbs, if desired.

NOTES:

- For extra flavor, drizzle with balsamic glaze or lemon juice.
- You can add other roasted vegetables, such as carrots or zucchini.
- Serve warm or cold as a side dish or main course.

NUTRITIONAL INFO (approximate per serving):

- Calories: 250-300 | Protein: 5-8 g | Fat: 5-8 g | Carbohydrates: 35-40 g | Sodium: 100-150 mg (may vary based on ingredients) | Potassium: 300-400 mg | Phosphorus: 150-200 mg

Quinoa Salad with Grilled Chicken or Tofu

This versatile salad is packed with protein and fiber, making it a satisfying and healthy meal option.

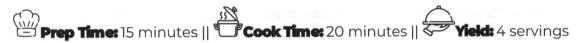 **Prep Time:** 15 minutes || **Cook Time:** 20 minutes || **Yield:** 4 servings

INGREDIENTS

- 1 cup quinoa, rinsed
- 2 cups vegetable broth
- 1/2 cup chopped cucumber
- 1/2 cup cherry tomatoes, halved
- 1/4 cup red onion, finely chopped
- 1/4 cup fresh parsley, chopped

- 2 tablespoons olive oil
- 1 tablespoon lemon juice
- 1/4 teaspoon garlic powder
- Salt and pepper to taste
- 4 oz grilled chicken breast or tofu, cubed (optional)

INSTRUCTIONS:

1. Rinse quinoa under cold water until water runs clear.

2. In a medium saucepan, combine quinoa and vegetable broth. Bring to a boil, then reduce heat, cover, and simmer for 15 minutes, or until liquid is absorbed.

3. Fluff quinoa with a fork and let cool completely.

4. In a large bowl, combine cooked quinoa, cucumber, cherry tomatoes, red onion, and parsley.

5. In a small bowl, whisk together olive oil, lemon juice, garlic powder, salt, and pepper.

6. Pour dressing over the quinoa mixture and toss to coat.

7. Stir in grilled chicken or tofu, if using.

NOTES:

- For a creamier salad, add a dollop of Greek yogurt or avocado.
- You can add other vegetables, such as bell peppers, or chickpeas for extra protein.

NUTRITIONAL INFO (approximate per serving):

- Calories: 250-300 | Protein: 15-20 g | Fat: 10-12 g | Carbohydrates: 30-35 g | Sodium: 100-150 mg (may vary based on ingredients) | Potassium: 300-400 mg | Phosphorus: 150-200 mg

Lentil Pasta with Tomato Sauce and Vegetables

This vegetarian-friendly dish is packed with protein and fiber.

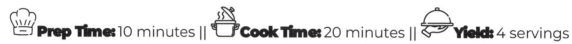 **Prep Time:** 10 minutes || **Cook Time:** 20 minutes || **Yield:** 4 servings

INGREDIENTS

- 8 oz lentil pasta

- 1 jar (24 ounces) low-sodium marinara sauce

- 1/2 onion, chopped

- 1 carrot, diced

- 1/2 green bell pepper, sliced

- 1 clove garlic, minced

- 1/4 cup chopped fresh basil

- Salt and pepper to taste

INSTRUCTIONS:

1. Cook lentil pasta. Drain and set aside.

2. In a large skillet, sauté onion, carrot, and green bell pepper in a bit of olive oil until softened. Add garlic and cook for 30 seconds more.

3. Stir in marinara sauce and bring to a simmer.

4. Add cooked lentil pasta to the sauce and toss to coat.

5. Simmer for a few minutes to allow flavors to blend. Stir in fresh basil and season with salt and pepper.

NOTES:

- For a creamier sauce, add a dollop of Greek yogurt or ricotta cheese.

- You can add other vegetables, such as mushrooms or zucchini, to the dish.

- Serve with a side salad or a sprinkle of Parmesan cheese for extra flavor.

NUTRITIONAL INFO (approximate per serving):

- Calories: 300-350 | Protein: 15-20 g | Fat: 5-8 g | Carbohydrates: 40-45 g | Sodium: 100-150 mg (may vary based on ingredients) | Potassium: 300-400 mg | Phosphorus: 150-200 mg

Shrimp Scampi Pasta

This classic Italian dish is a flavorful and satisfying meal.

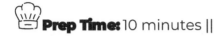**Prep Time:** 10 minutes || 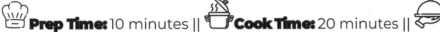**Cook Time:** 20 minutes || 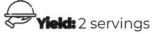**Yield:** 2 servings

INGREDIENTS

- 8 oz shrimp, peeled and deveined
- 8 oz whole-wheat pasta
- 2 cloves garlic, minced
- 1/4 cup dry white wine (optional)
- 1/4 cup low-sodium chicken broth
- 2 tablespoons fresh lemon juice

- 2 tablespoons capers, drained
- 1/4 teaspoon red pepper flakes (optional)
- 1/4 cup fresh parsley, chopped
- Olive oil
- Salt and pepper to taste

INSTRUCTIONS:

1. Cook pasta. Drain, reserving 1/4 cup pasta water.

2. In a large skillet, heat olive oil over medium-high heat. Add shrimp and cook until pink and opaque. Remove from skillet and set aside.

3. Add garlic to the skillet and cook for 30 seconds, being careful not to burn.

4. Stir in white wine (if using) and chicken broth. Bring to a simmer.

5. Return shrimp to the skillet and add lemon juice, capers, and red pepper flakes (if using). Cook for 1-2 minutes, or until shrimp is heated through.

6. Add cooked pasta and reserved pasta water to the skillet. Toss to coat.

7. Stir in parsley and season with salt and pepper. Serve immediately.

NOTES:

- You can substitute shrimp with other seafood, such as scallops or clams.
- Serve with a side salad for a more balanced meal.

NUTRITIONAL INFO (approximate per serving):

- Calories: 400-450 | Protein: 25-30 g | Fat: 10-12 g | Carbohydrates: 50-60 g | Sodium: 100-150 mg (may vary based on ingredients) | Potassium: 200-300 mg | Phosphorus: 150-200 mg

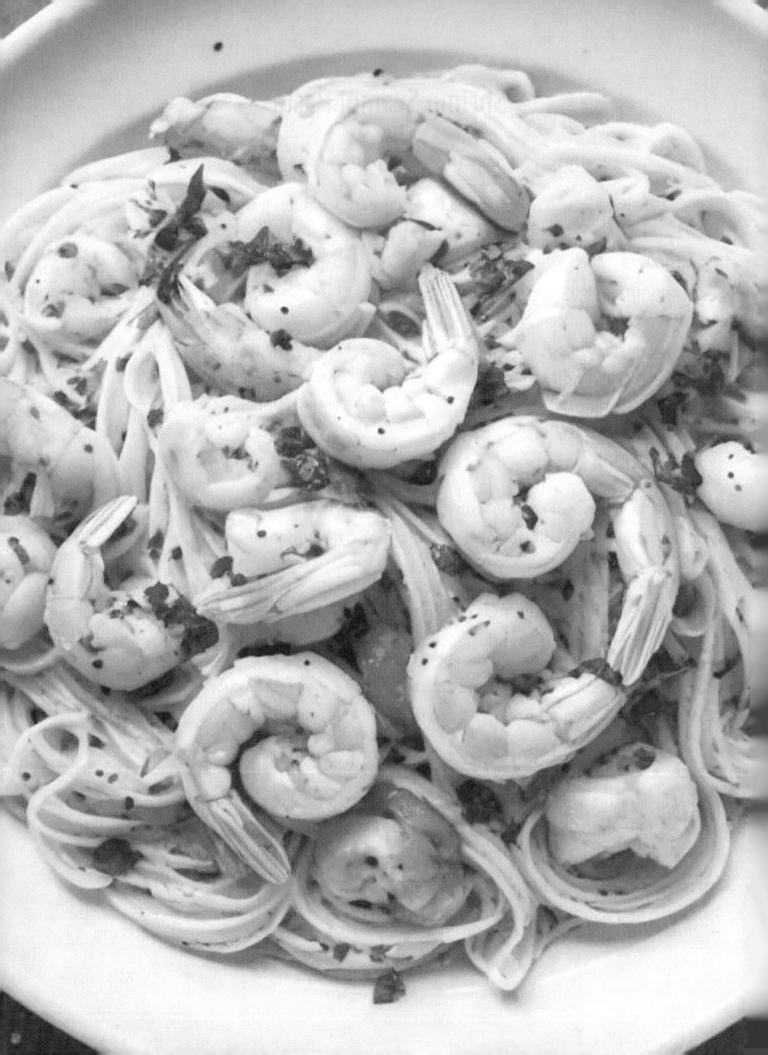

Whole-Wheat Penne with Marinara Sauce and Meatballs

This classic Italian dish can be adapted to fit a diabetic and renal diet by using whole-wheat pasta, low-sodium ingredients, and lean meatballs.

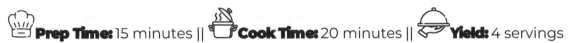 **Prep Time:** 15 minutes || **Cook Time:** 20 minutes || **Yield:** 4 servings

INGREDIENTS

- 8 oz whole-wheat penne pasta

- 1 jar (24 ounces) low-sodium marinara sauce

- 1 pound lean ground turkey or chicken

- 1/2 cup bread crumbs (low-sodium)

- 1/4 cup onion, finely chopped

- 1 egg white

- 1/4 teaspoon garlic powder

- 1/4 teaspoon dried oregano

- Salt and pepper to taste

- Optional: grated Parmesan cheese (low-sodium)

INSTRUCTIONS:

1. Preheat oven to 375°F (190°C).

2. Cook pasta. Drain and set aside.

3. In a large bowl, combine ground turkey or chicken, bread crumbs, onion, egg white, garlic powder, oregano, salt, and pepper. Shape into meatballs.

4. In a large skillet, brown meatballs on all sides. Remove from skillet and set aside.

5. In the same skillet, heat marinara sauce.

6. Combine cooked pasta and meatballs with marinara sauce in a large bowl.

7. Serve immediately, topped with grated Parmesan cheese if desired.

NOTES:

- For a thicker sauce, simmer the marinara sauce for a few minutes before adding the pasta and meatballs.

- You can substitute ground turkey or chicken with lean ground beef or pork.

NUTRITIONAL INFO (approximate per serving):

- Calories: 400-450 | Protein: 25-30 g | Fat: 10-12 g | Carbohydrates: 50-60 g | Sodium: 100-150 mg (may vary based on ingredients) | Potassium: 300-400 mg | Phosphorus: 150-200 mg

Pesto Pasta with Grilled Chicken or Salmon

This dish offers a flavorful and satisfying meal, packed with protein and healthy fats.

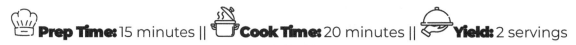 **Prep Time:** 15 minutes || **Cook Time:** 20 minutes || **Yield:** 2 servings

INGREDIENTS

- 8 oz whole-wheat pasta
- 1/2 cup pesto (low-sodium)
- 4 oz grilled chicken breast or salmon, sliced
- 1/4 cup grated Parmesan cheese (low-sodium)
- Salt and pepper to taste

INSTRUCTIONS:

1. Cook pasta. Drain, reserving 1/4 cup pasta water.

2. In a large skillet, combine cooked pasta, pesto, and reserved pasta water. Stir until pesto is melted and coats the pasta.

3. Add grilled chicken or salmon to the pasta and toss to combine.

4. Stir in Parmesan cheese and season with salt and pepper.

NOTES:

- For a creamier sauce, add a dollop of Greek yogurt or ricotta cheese.
- You can add other vegetables, such as roasted cherry tomatoes or sautéed spinach, to the pasta.
- Serve immediately for the best flavor.

NUTRITIONAL INFO (approximate per serving):

- Calories: 500-600 | Protein: 30-35 g | Fat: 20-25 g | Carbohydrates: 50-60 g | Sodium: 100-150 mg (may vary based on ingredients) | Potassium: 300-400 mg | Phosphorus: 150-200 mg

VEGETABLE DISHES

Mediterranean Chickpea Salad

This vibrant and flavorful salad is packed with protein and fiber.

**Prep Time:** 15 minutes || **Cook Time:** 0 minutes || **Yield:** 4 servings

INGREDIENTS

- 1 can (15 ounces) chickpeas, drained and rinsed
- 1 cucumber, diced
- 1 red bell pepper, diced
- 1/2 red onion, finely chopped
- 1/4 cup chopped fresh parsley
- 1/4 cup crumbled feta cheese (low-sodium)
- 2 tablespoons olive oil
- 1 tablespoon lemon juice
- 1/2 teaspoon dried oregano
- Salt and pepper to taste

INSTRUCTIONS:

1. In a large bowl, combine chickpeas, cucumber, red bell pepper, red onion, and parsley.

2. In a small bowl, whisk together olive oil, lemon juice, oregano, salt, and pepper.

3. Pour dressing over the salad and toss to coat.

4. Crumble feta cheese over the salad and serve immediately.

NOTES:

- For a crunchier salad, add chopped celery or a handful of toasted pine nuts.
- You can adjust the acidity by adding more or less lemon juice.
- Serve over a bed of greens or as a side dish.

NUTRITIONAL INFO (approximate per serving):

- Calories: 250-300 | Protein: 10-12 g | Fat: 10-12 g | Carbohydrates: 25-30 g | Sodium: 100-150 mg (may vary based on ingredients) | Potassium: 300-400 mg | Phosphorus: 150-200 mg

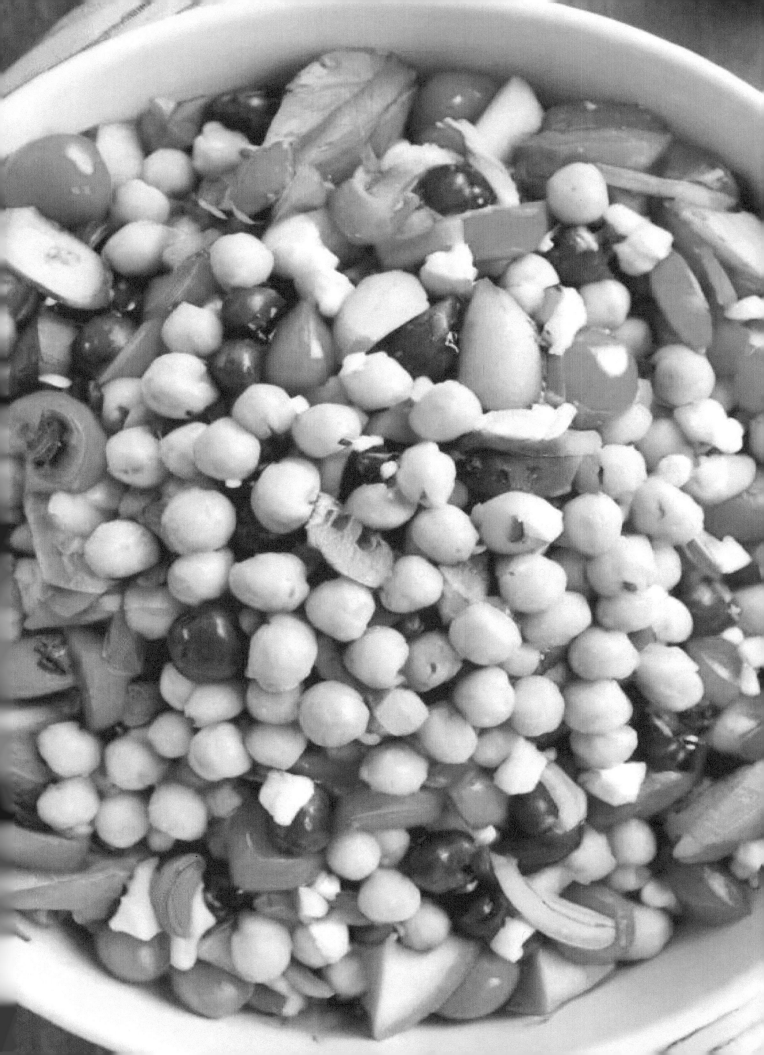

Lentil Loaf

While a traditional lentil loaf might take longer to prepare, this recipe offers a quicker, lighter version suitable for a diabetic and renal diet.

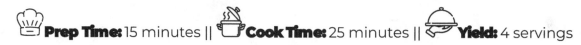 **Prep Time:** 15 minutes || **Cook Time:** 25 minutes || **Yield:** 4 servings

INGREDIENTS

- 1 can (15 ounces) green lentils, rinsed and drained

- 1/2 cup cooked brown rice

- 1/2 cup grated carrot

- 1/4 cup onion, finely chopped

- 1 egg white

- 1/4 cup bread crumbs (low-sodium)

- 1 teaspoon dried thyme

- 1/2 teaspoon garlic powder

- Salt and pepper to taste

INSTRUCTIONS:

1. Preheat oven to 375°F (190°C).

2. In a large bowl, combine lentils, brown rice, carrot, onion, egg white, bread crumbs, thyme, garlic powder, salt, and pepper. Mix well.

3. Transfer the mixture to a loaf pan and shape into a loaf.

4. Bake for 25 minutes, or until firm and golden brown.

NOTES:

- Serve with a side of steamed vegetables or a green salad.

- For extra flavor, add chopped fresh herbs like parsley or dill.

- You can use a food processor to pulse the ingredients for a smoother texture.

NUTRITIONAL INFO (approximate per serving):

- Calories: 200-250 | Protein: 15-20 g | Fat: 5-8 g | Carbohydrates: 30-35 g | Sodium: 100-150 mg (may vary based on ingredients) | Potassium: 300-400 mg | Phosphorus: 150-200 mg

Tofu Scramble

This plant-based protein-packed dish is a great alternative to traditional egg scrambles.

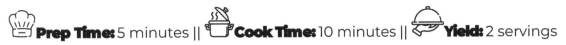 **Prep Time:** 5 minutes || **Cook Time:** 10 minutes || **Yield:** 2 servings

INGREDIENTS

- 1 block extra-firm tofu, crumbled
- 1/4 onion, chopped
- 1/4 green bell pepper, chopped
- 1 clove garlic, minced
- 1 tablespoon olive oil
- Salt and pepper to taste
- Optional: spinach, tomatoes, or other vegetables

INSTRUCTIONS:

1. Squeeze out excess water from the crumbled tofu using paper towels.

2. Heat olive oil in a large skillet over medium heat. Add onion and green bell pepper, cook until softened.

3. Stir in garlic and cook for 30 seconds, or until fragrant.

4. Add crumbled tofu to the skillet and break it up with a spatula.

5. Season with salt and pepper. Cook until heated through and golden brown.

6. Stir in spinach or other desired vegetables.

NOTES:

- For extra flavor, add a sprinkle of nutritional yeast or a squeeze of lemon juice.
- Serve with whole-grain toast or a side of avocado for a complete meal.
- You can customize this recipe by adding your favorite spices or herbs.

NUTRITIONAL INFO (approximate per serving):

- Calories: 150-200 | Protein: 10-12 g | Fat: 5-8 g | Carbohydrates: 5-10 g | Sodium: 100-150 mg (may vary based on ingredients) | Potassium: 200-300 mg | Phosphorus: 100-150 mg

Chickpea Curry

This hearty and flavorful curry is a great plant-based protein option.

 **Prep Time:** 10 minutes || **Cook Time:** 20 minutes || **Yield:** 4 servings

INGREDIENTS

- 1 tablespoon olive oil
- 1 onion, chopped
- 1 green bell pepper, chopped
- 1 clove garlic, minced
- 1 teaspoon ground cumin
- 1 teaspoon ground coriander
- 1/2 teaspoon turmeric

- 1 can (15 ounces) chickpeas, drained and rinsed
- 1 can (14.5 ounces) diced tomatoes, undrained
- 1 cup vegetable broth
- Fresh cilantro, for garnish
- Salt and pepper to taste

INSTRUCTIONS:

1. Heat olive oil in a large pot or Dutch oven over medium heat. Add onion and green bell pepper, cook until softened.

2. Stir in garlic, cumin, coriander, and turmeric. Cook for 30 seconds, or until fragrant.

3. Add chickpeas, diced tomatoes, and vegetable broth to the pot. Bring to a simmer.

4. Reduce heat and simmer for 15-20 minutes, or until the sauce has thickened.

5. Season with salt and pepper to taste.

6. Garnish with fresh cilantro before serving.

NOTES:

- Serve with brown rice or whole-wheat naan for a complete meal.
- You can adjust the spice level by adding red pepper flakes or cayenne pepper.
- For a creamier curry, stir in a dollop of Greek yogurt or coconut milk before serving.

NUTRITIONAL INFO (approximate per serving):

- Calories: 250-300 | Protein: 15-20 g | Fat: 5-8 g | Carbohydrates: 30-35 g | Sodium: 100-150 mg (may vary based on ingredients) | Potassium: 300-400 mg | Phosphorus: 150-200 mg

Vegetable Burger

This hearty and flavorful burger is a great plant-based option.

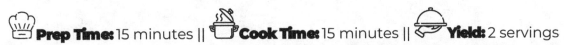

Prep Time: 15 minutes || **Cook Time:** 15 minutes || **Yield:** 2 servings

INGREDIENTS

- 1 cup cooked brown rice
- 1 can black beans, rinsed and drained
- 1/2 onion, finely chopped
- 1 carrot, grated
- 1/4 cup bread crumbs
- 1 egg white
- 1 teaspoon cumin
- 1/2 teaspoon chili powder
- Salt and pepper to taste

INSTRUCTIONS:

1. In a large bowl, combine brown rice, black beans, onion, carrot, bread crumbs, egg white, cumin, chili powder, salt, and pepper.

2. Shape the mixture into two burger patties.

3. Heat a large skillet over medium heat with a drizzle of olive oil.

4. Cook burgers for 5-7 minutes per side, or until golden brown and cooked through.

NOTES:

- Serve on whole-grain buns with your favorite low-sodium condiments.
- You can add other vegetables to the burger patties, such as zucchini or corn.
- For a gluten-free option, use gluten-free bread crumbs.

NUTRITIONAL INFO (approximate per serving):

- Calories: 250-300 | Protein: 15-20 g | Fat: 5-8 g | Carbohydrates: 30-35 g | Sodium: 100-150 mg (may vary based on ingredients) | Potassium: 300-400 mg | Phosphorus: 150-200 mg

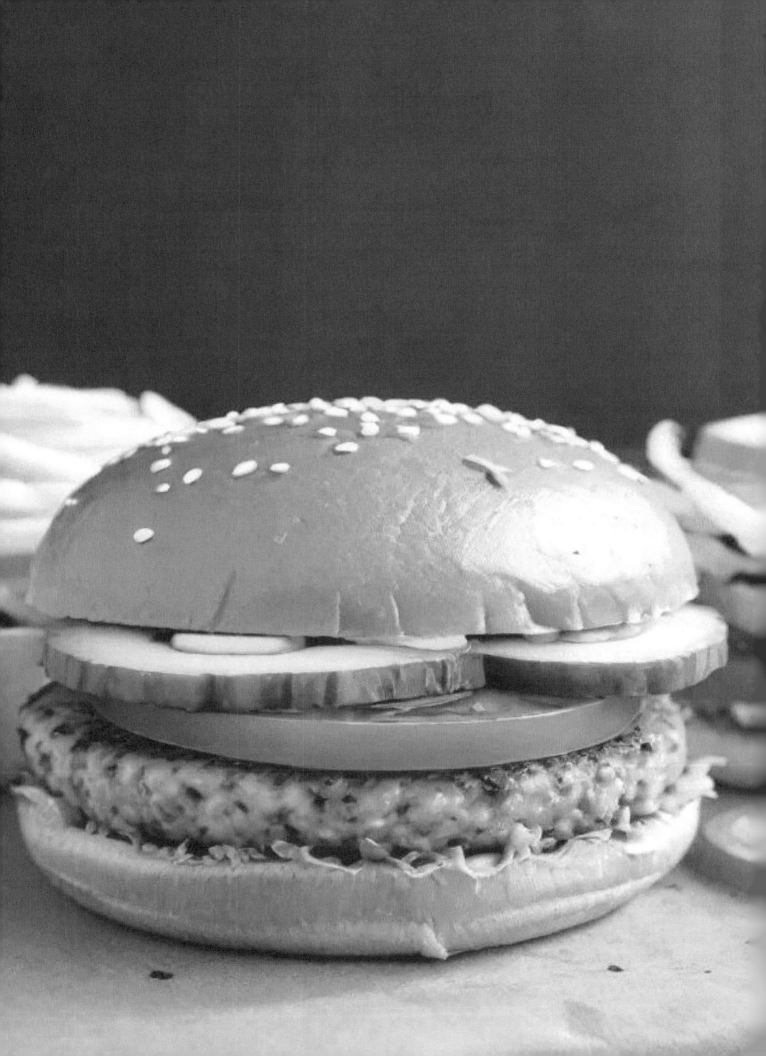

Vegetable Stir-Fry

This dish is a quick and healthy option, packed with nutrients and low in calories.

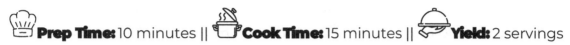 **Prep Time:** 10 minutes || **Cook Time:** 15 minutes || **Yield:** 2 servings

INGREDIENTS

- 1 tablespoon olive oil
- 1/2 onion, sliced
- 1 green bell pepper, sliced
- 1 carrot, sliced
- 1/2 cup broccoli florets
- 2 cloves garlic, minced
- 1 teaspoon low-sodium soy sauce
- 1/4 teaspoon red pepper flakes (optional)

INSTRUCTIONS:

1. Heat olive oil in a large skillet or wok over medium-high heat.

2. Add onion and green bell pepper, cook until softened.

3. Add carrot and broccoli, cook for 2-3 minutes, or until slightly tender.

4. Stir in garlic and cook for 30 seconds.

5. Season with soy sauce and red pepper flakes (if using).

6. Serve immediately over brown rice or quinoa.

NOTES:

- For extra flavor, add a splash of rice vinegar or sesame oil.

- You can substitute or add other vegetables, such as snap peas, mushrooms, or water chestnuts.

- Serve with a side of tofu or lean protein for a more complete meal.

NUTRITIONAL INFO (approximate per serving):

- Calories: 150-200 | Protein: 3-5 g | Fat: 5-8 g | Carbohydrates: 10-15 g | Sodium: 100-150 mg (may vary based on ingredients) | Potassium: 200-300 mg | Phosphorus: 100-150 mg

Vegetable Primavera

This vibrant dish is packed with nutrients and low in calories.

 **Prep Time:** 10 minutes || **Cook Time:** 15 minutes || **Yield:** 4 servings

INGREDIENTS

- 1 tablespoon olive oil
- 1 onion, chopped
- 2 cloves garlic, minced
- 2 carrots, sliced
- 1 zucchini, sliced
- 1 red bell pepper, sliced
- 1 cup broccoli florets
- 1/4 cup low-sodium vegetable broth
- 1/4 teaspoon dried oregano
- 1/4 teaspoon dried basil
- Salt and pepper to taste

INSTRUCTIONS:

1. Heat olive oil in a large skillet over medium heat. Add onion and garlic, cook until softened.

2. Stir in carrots, zucchini, and bell pepper. Cook for 5-7 minutes, or until slightly tender.

3. Add broccoli and vegetable broth to the skillet. Bring to a simmer.

4. Season with oregano, basil, salt, and pepper. Cook for an additional 5 minutes, or until broccoli is tender.

NOTES:

- Serve over whole-grain pasta or brown rice for a more filling meal.
- You can add other vegetables, such as mushrooms, spinach, or snap peas.
- For extra flavor, top with a sprinkle of Parmesan cheese or a squeeze of lemon juice.

NUTRITIONAL INFO (approximate per serving):

- Calories: 150-200 | Protein: 3-5 g | Fat: 5-8 g | Carbohydrates: 10-15 g | Sodium: 100-150 mg (may vary based on ingredients) | Potassium: 200-300 mg | Phosphorus: 100-150 mg

Kidney Bean Burger

These hearty and flavorful kidney bean burgers are packed with protein and fiber, making them a satisfying and healthy option for individuals with diabetes and kidney disease.

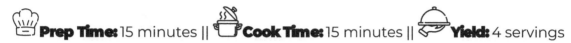 **Prep Time:** 15 minutes || **Cook Time:** 15 minutes || **Yield:** 4 servings

INGREDIENTS

- 1 can (15 ounces) kidney beans, rinsed and drained

- 1/2 cup cooked brown rice

- 1/4 cup finely chopped onion

- 1 clove garlic, minced

- 1/4 cup bread crumbs

- 1 egg white

- 1 tablespoon olive oil

- 1 teaspoon ground cumin

- 1/2 teaspoon chili powder

- Salt and pepper to taste

- Low-sodium bun (optional)

- Low-sodium condiments (optional)

INSTRUCTIONS

1. In a large bowl, combine kidney beans, brown rice, onion, garlic, bread crumbs, egg white, olive oil, cumin, chili powder, salt, and pepper. Mash the mixture together until it forms a cohesive patty consistency.

2. Divide the mixture into four equal parts and shape them into patties.

3. Heat a large skillet over medium heat. Cook the patties for about 5-7 minutes per side, or until golden brown and cooked through.

4. Serve on a low-sodium bun with your favorite low-sodium condiments, if desired.

NOTES

- For a gluten-free option, use gluten-free bread crumbs.

- To reduce sodium content, use fresh garlic and onion instead of pre-minced or chopped varieties.

- Serve with a side of steamed vegetables for a complete meal.

NUTRITIONAL INFO (approximate per serving):

- Calories: 200-250 | Protein: 15-20 g | Fat: 5-8 g | Carbohydrates: 25-30 g | Sodium: 100-150 mg (may vary based on ingredients) | Potassium: 300-400 mg | Phosphorus: 150-200 mg

Green Beans with Red Pepper and Garlic

This simple yet flavorful side dish is packed with vitamins, minerals, and fiber. Green beans are a low-sodium vegetable, making them an excellent choice for a renal diet.

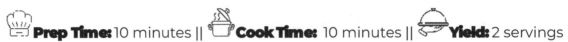

Prep Time: 10 minutes || **Cook Time:** 10 minutes || **Yield:** 2 servings

INGREDIENTS

- 1 pound fresh green beans, trimmed
- 1 red bell pepper, sliced
- 2 cloves garlic, minced
- 1 tablespoon olive oil
- Salt and pepper to taste

INSTRUCTIONS

1. Bring a large pot of salted water to a boil.

2. Add green beans and cook for 3-4 minutes, or until tender-crisp. Drain.

3. Heat olive oil in a large skillet over medium heat. Add garlic and cook for 30 seconds, or until fragrant.

4. Add red bell pepper and cook for 2-3 minutes, or until softened.

5. Add cooked green beans to the skillet and stir-fry for 2 minutes, or until heated through.

6. Season with salt and pepper to taste. Serve immediately.

NOTES

- For a milder flavor, use less garlic.
- You can substitute red bell pepper with yellow or orange bell pepper.
- Serve as a side dish or as a main course with a protein source.
- Stir in a tablespoon of grated Parmesan cheese (monitor sodium intake).
- Serve with a dollop of plain Greek yogurt for a creamy sauce.

NUTRITIONAL INFO (per serving):

- Calories: 50 | Protein: 2g | Fat: 3g | Carbohydrates: 7g | Sodium: 10mg | Potassium: 300mg | Phosphorus: 50mg

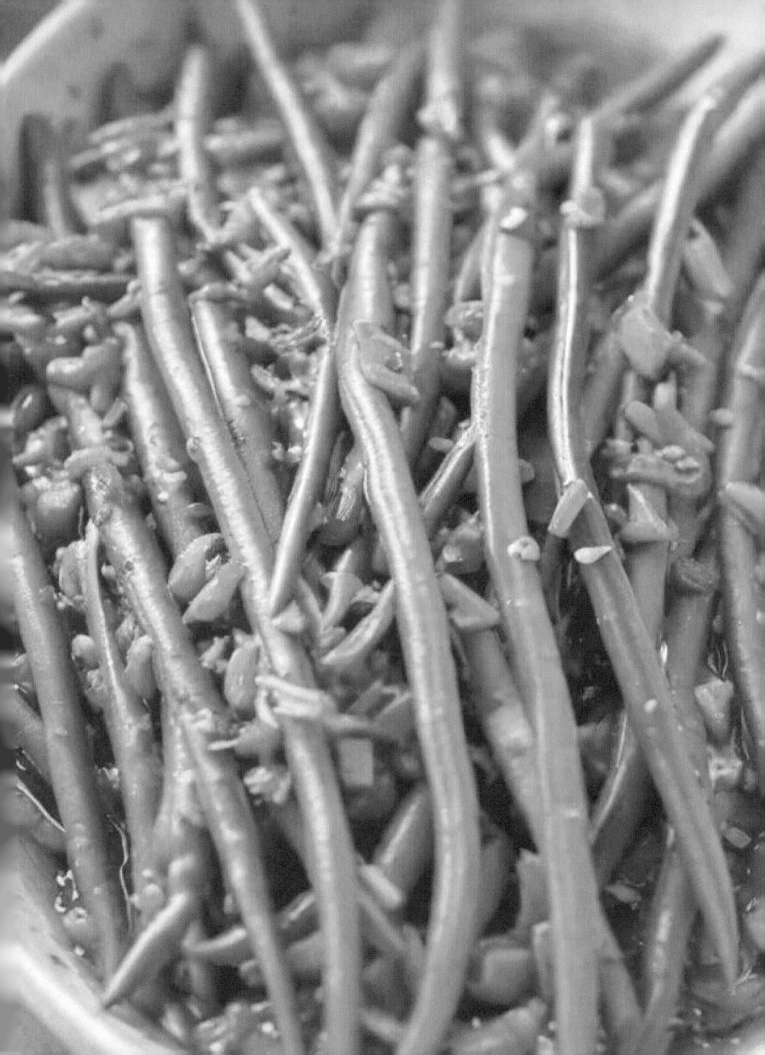

Broccoli with Garlic and Lemon

This simple yet flavorful side dish is packed with vitamins, minerals, and fiber. Broccoli is a low-sodium vegetable, making it an excellent choice for a renal diet.

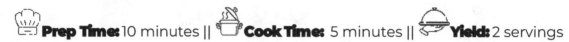 **Prep Time:** 10 minutes || **Cook Time:** 5 minutes || **Yield:** 2 servings

INGREDIENTS

- 1 head broccoli, cut into florets
- 2 cloves garlic, minced
- 1 tablespoon olive oil
- 1 tablespoon lemon juice
- Salt and pepper to taste

INSTRUCTIONS

1. Bring a large pot of salted water to a boil.

2. Add broccoli florets to the boiling water and cook for 3-4 minutes, or until tender-crisp.

3. Drain the broccoli and transfer to a bowl.

4. In a small skillet, heat olive oil over medium heat. Add garlic and cook for 30 seconds, or until fragrant.

5. Pour the garlic and olive oil over the cooked broccoli.

6. Squeeze lemon juice over the broccoli and season with salt and pepper to taste.

7. Toss to combine. Serve immediately.

NOTES

- For a milder flavor, use less garlic.
- You can add a squeeze of fresh orange juice for a different flavor profile.
- Serve as a side dish or as a main course with a protein source.

NUTRITIONAL INFO (per serving):

- Calories: 50 | Protein: 3g | Fat: 3g | Carbohydrates: 7g | Sodium: 10mg | Potassium: 300mg | Phosphorus: 60mg

White Bean Dip

This creamy and flavorful dip is a perfect appetizer or snack. White beans provide a good source of plant-based protein, while the fresh herbs add a burst of flavor.

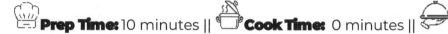 **Prep Time:** 10 minutes || **Cook Time:** 0 minutes || **Yield:** 2 servings

INGREDIENTS

- 1 can (15 ounces) white beans, rinsed and drained

- 3 tablespoons extra-virgin olive oil

- 2 cloves garlic, minced

- 2 tablespoons fresh lemon juice

- 1/4 cup chopped fresh parsley

- 1/4 cup chopped fresh dill

- Salt and pepper to taste

- Pita bread or vegetable sticks, for serving

INSTRUCTIONS

1. In a food processor, combine white beans, olive oil, garlic, lemon juice, parsley, and dill.

2. Process until smooth and creamy, scraping down the sides of the food processor as needed.

3. Season with salt and pepper to taste.

4. Serve with pita bread or vegetable sticks.

NOTES

- For a thicker dip, add less lemon juice.

- You can adjust the herbs to your taste preference.

- Serve with whole-grain crackers for a crunchy texture.

NUTRITIONAL INFO (per serving):

- Calories: 200 | Protein: 8g | Fat: 10g | Carbohydrates: 20g | Sodium: 100mg | Potassium: 400mg | Phosphorus: 120mg

Pickled Asparagus

Pickled asparagus is a tangy and flavorful side dish or snack. This recipe uses a low-sodium pickling brine for those following a renal diet.

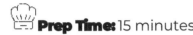**Prep Time:** 15 minutes || 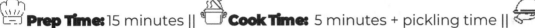**Cook Time:** 5 minutes + pickling time || 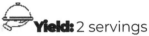**Yield:** 2 servings

INGREDIENTS

- 1 pound fresh asparagus, trimmed

- 1 cup white vinegar

- 1 cup water

- 1 tablespoon sugar substitute (optional)

- 1 teaspoon mustard seeds

- 1/2 teaspoon red pepper flakes (optional)

- 1 bay leaf

INSTRUCTIONS

1. Bring a large pot of salted water to a boil. Add asparagus and cook for 2-3 minutes, or until tender-crisp. Drain immediately.

2. In a clean glass jar, combine vinegar, water, sugar substitute (if using), mustard seeds, red pepper flakes, and bay leaf.

3. Pack the cooked asparagus tightly into the jar.

4. Pour the pickling brine over the asparagus, ensuring it covers all the spears.

5. Seal the jar tightly and let it cool to room temperature before refrigerating.

6. The asparagus will be ready to eat in at least 24 hours.

NOTES

- For a milder flavor, omit the red pepper flakes.

- Adjust the amount of sugar substitute to your taste preference.

- Store the pickled asparagus in the refrigerator for up to two weeks.

NUTRITIONAL INFO (per serving):

- Calories: 20 | Protein: 2g | Fat: 0g | Carbohydrates: 3g | Sodium: 100mg | Potassium: 200mg | Phosphorus: 50mg

BREAKFAST

Greek Yogurt with Berries

This simple yet refreshing snack is packed with protein and antioxidants.

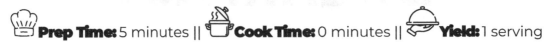 **Prep Time:** 5 minutes || **Cook Time:** 0 minutes || **Yield:** 1 serving

INGREDIENTS

- 1/2 cup Greek yogurt (plain or low-fat)
- 1/2 cup mixed berries (blueberries, raspberries, strawberries)
- Optional: honey or maple syrup (use sparingly)
- Optional: granola or nuts

INSTRUCTIONS:

1. In a bowl, combine Greek yogurt and mixed berries.

2. Drizzle with honey or maple syrup, if desired.

3. Top with granola or nuts for added crunch and texture.

NOTES:

- Choose a Greek yogurt that is low in sodium and added sugars.
- For a lower-calorie option, use fresh or frozen berries.
- Experiment with different types of berries and toppings to create your own flavor combinations.

NUTRITIONAL INFO (approximate per serving):

- Calories: 100-150 | Protein: 10-12 g | Fat: 2-4 g | Carbohydrates: 10-15 g | Sodium: 100-150 mg (may vary based on ingredients) | Potassium: 200-300 mg | Phosphorus: 100-150 mg

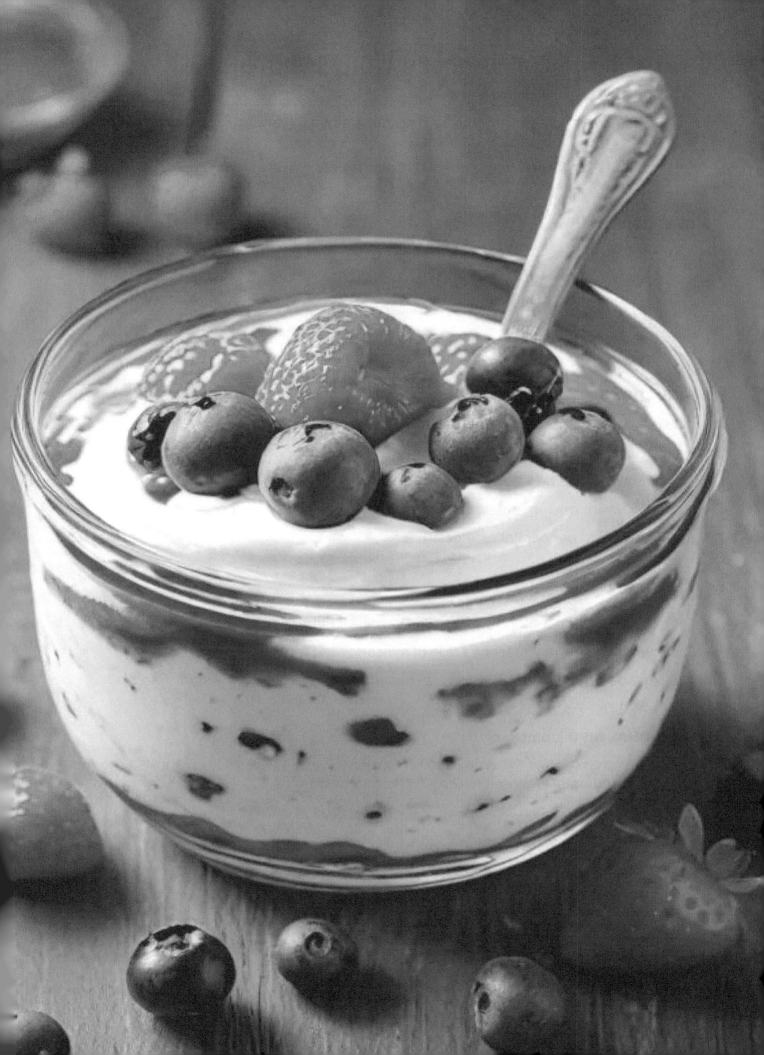

Scrambled Egg Whites with Spinach

This low-calorie, protein-packed option is a healthy and quick breakfast choice.

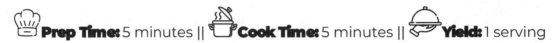 **Prep Time:** 5 minutes || **Cook Time:** 5 minutes || **Yield:** 1 serving

INGREDIENTS

- 2 egg whites
- 1/4 cup fresh spinach, chopped
- Salt and pepper to taste
- Optional: red pepper flakes

INSTRUCTIONS:

1. In a small bowl, whisk together egg whites, salt, and pepper.
2. Heat a non-stick skillet over medium heat.
3. Add spinach to the skillet and cook until wilted.
4. Pour egg white mixture into the skillet and scramble gently until cooked through.
5. Season with red pepper flakes, if desired.

NOTES:

- For extra flavor, add a sprinkle of grated Parmesan cheese or a squeeze of lemon juice.
- Serve with whole-grain toast or a side of avocado for a more complete meal.
- You can add other vegetables, such as mushrooms or onions, to the scramble.

NUTRITIONAL INFO (approximate per serving):

- Calories: 50-70 | Protein: 7-9 g | Fat: 1-2 g | Carbohydrates: 1-2 g | Sodium: 100-150 mg (may vary based on ingredients) | Potassium: 200-300 mg | Phosphorus: 100-150 mg

Oatmeal with Apples

This classic breakfast option is a healthy and satisfying way to start your day.

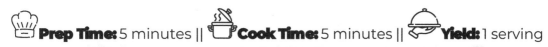 **Prep Time:** 5 minutes || **Cook Time:** 5 minutes || **Yield:** 1 serving

INGREDIENTS

- 1/2 cup rolled oats
- 1 cup water
- Pinch of salt
- 1/2 apple, diced
- Cinnamon (optional)

INSTRUCTIONS:

1. In a small saucepan, combine oats, water, and salt.
2. Bring to a boil, then reduce heat and simmer for 5 minutes, or until desired consistency.
3. Stir in diced apple.
4. Sprinkle with cinnamon, if desired.

NOTES:

- For a creamier oatmeal, add a splash of milk or plant-based milk.
- Top with a sprinkle of nuts or seeds for added texture and protein.
- Use unsweetened apple sauce as a topping for a different flavor profile.

NUTRITIONAL INFO (approximate per serving):

- Calories: 150-200 | Protein: 5-7 g | Fat: 2-4 g | Carbohydrates: 25-30 g | Sodium: 100-150 mg (may vary based on ingredients) | Potassium: 200-300 mg | Phosphorus: 100-150 mg

Egg Salad

This classic protein-packed spread is a versatile option for sandwiches, wraps, or a standalone snack.

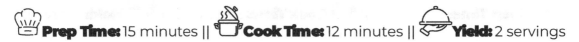 **Prep Time:** 15 minutes || **Cook Time:** 12 minutes || **Yield:** 2 servings

INGREDIENTS

- 4 large eggs
- 1/4 cup low-fat mayonnaise
- 1 teaspoon Dijon mustard
- 1/4 celery stalk, finely chopped
- 1/4 red onion, finely chopped
- Salt and pepper to taste

INSTRUCTIONS:

1. Place eggs in a saucepan and cover with cold water. Bring to a boil, then reduce heat and simmer for 10 minutes.

2. Transfer eggs to an ice bath to cool rapidly. Peel and chop eggs.

3. In a medium bowl, combine chopped eggs, mayonnaise, Dijon mustard, celery, and red onion.

4. Season with salt and pepper to taste.

NOTES:

- For extra flavor, add a squeeze of lemon juice or a sprinkle of dried dill.
- Serve on whole-grain bread, crackers, or as a filling for lettuce wraps.
- You can adjust the consistency by adding more or less mayonnaise.

NUTRITIONAL INFO (approximate per serving):

- Calories: 200-250 | Protein: 15-20 g | Fat: 10-12 g | Carbohydrates: 5-10 g | Sodium: 100-150 mg (may vary based on ingredients) | Potassium: 200-300 mg | Phosphorus: 100-150 mg

Cottage Cheese with Pineapple

This simple yet refreshing snack is packed with protein and nutrients.

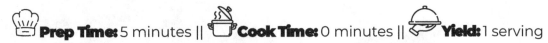 **Prep Time:** 5 minutes || **Cook Time:** 0 minutes || **Yield:** 1 serving

INGREDIENTS

- 1/2 cup low-fat cottage cheese
- 1/4 cup pineapple chunks (fresh or canned, drained)
- Optional: sprinkle of cinnamon

INSTRUCTIONS:

1. In a bowl, combine cottage cheese and pineapple chunks.
2. Stir gently to combine.
3. Sprinkle with cinnamon, if desired.

NOTES:

- For added flavor, you can add a squeeze of lime or lemon juice.
- For a crunchier texture, add a handful of chopped nuts or seeds.
- Serve chilled for a refreshing snack.

NUTRITIONAL INFO (approximate per serving):

- Calories: 100-150 | Protein: 12-15 g | Fat: 2-4 g | Carbohydrates: 5-10 g | Sodium: 100-150 mg (may vary based on ingredients) | Potassium: 200-300 mg | Phosphorus: 100-150 mg

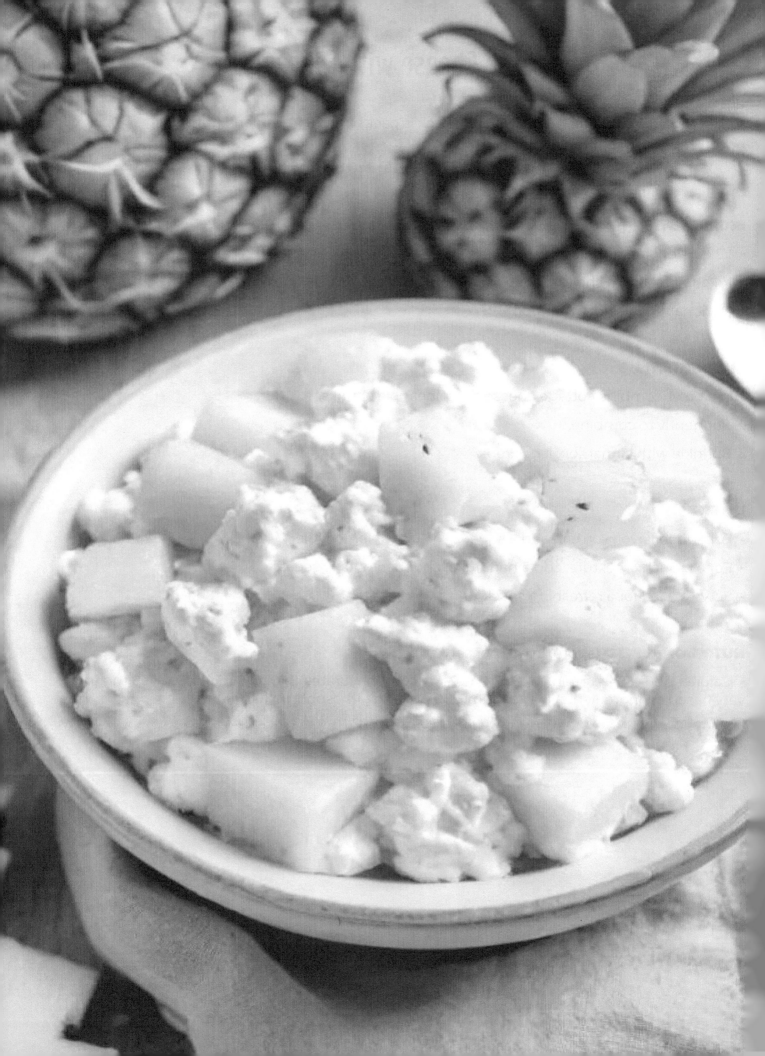

Whole-Grain Toast with Almond Butter

This simple yet satisfying breakfast option is packed with healthy fats and protein.

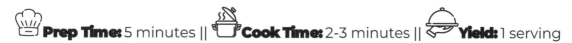 **Prep Time:** 5 minutes || **Cook Time:** 2-3 minutes || **Yield:** 1 serving

INGREDIENTS

- 1 slice whole-grain bread
- 1 tablespoon almond butter
- Optional toppings: sliced banana, chia seeds, cinnamon

INSTRUCTIONS:

1. Toast the whole-grain bread to your desired level of crispiness.
2. Spread almond butter evenly on the toast.
3. Add desired toppings, such as sliced banana, chia seeds, or cinnamon.

NOTES:

- Choose a whole-grain bread with a high fiber content.
- For a lower-calorie option, use a reduced-fat almond butter.
- Experiment with different toppings to create your own flavor combinations.

NUTRITIONAL INFO (approximate per serving):

- Calories: 200-250 | Protein: 7-9 g | Fat: 12-15 g | Carbohydrates: 20-25 g | Sodium: 100-150 mg (may vary based on ingredients) | Potassium: 200-300 mg | Phosphorus: 100-150 mg

Overnight Chia Seed Pudding

This healthy and versatile breakfast option can be customized with various toppings and flavorings.

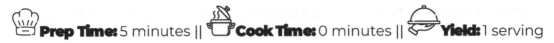 **Prep Time:** 5 minutes || **Cook Time:** 0 minutes || **Yield:** 1 serving

INGREDIENTS

- 3 tablespoons chia seeds
- 1 cup unsweetened almond milk (or other plant-based milk)
- 1 tablespoon maple syrup (or other sweetener)
- Pinch of salt
- Optional toppings: fresh berries, nuts, seeds, granola

INSTRUCTIONS:

1. In a jar or airtight container, combine chia seeds, almond milk, maple syrup, and salt.

2. Stir well to combine and remove any clumps.

3. Cover and refrigerate overnight, or for at least 4 hours.

4. In the morning, stir the pudding again.

5. Top with your desired toppings.

NOTES:

- For a thicker pudding, use less liquid.
- Experiment with different flavors by adding extracts like vanilla or almond.
- You can also add Greek yogurt for a creamier texture and extra protein.

NUTRITIONAL INFO (approximate per serving):

- Calories: 150-200 | Protein: 3-5 g | Fat: 5-8 g | Carbohydrates: 15-20 g | Sodium: 100-150 mg (may vary based on ingredients) | Potassium: 200-300 mg | Phosphorus: 100-150 mg

Avocado Toast

This simple yet satisfying dish is packed with healthy fats and fiber.

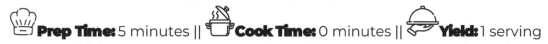 **Prep Time:** 5 minutes || **Cook Time:** 0 minutes || **Yield:** 1 serving

INGREDIENTS

- 1 slice whole-grain bread
- 1/2 ripe avocado, mashed
- 1/4 red onion, thinly sliced
- 1/4 cup cherry tomatoes, halved
- 1 tablespoon fresh cilantro, chopped
- Red pepper flakes (optional)
- Salt and pepper to taste

INSTRUCTIONS:

1. Toast the whole-grain bread to your desired level of crispiness.

2. Spread the mashed avocado evenly on the toast.

3. Top with thinly sliced red onion, halved cherry tomatoes, and chopped cilantro.

4. Sprinkle with red pepper flakes and season with salt and pepper to taste.

NOTES:

- For extra protein, add a sliced hard-boiled egg on top.

- You can experiment with different toppings, such as smoked salmon, feta cheese, or a drizzle of balsamic vinegar.

- Use whole-grain or sprouted bread for added fiber.

NUTRITIONAL INFO (approximate per serving):

- Calories: 200-250 | Protein: 3-5 g | Fat: 10-12 g | Carbohydrates: 20-25 g | Sodium: 100-150 mg (may vary based on ingredients) | Potassium: 300-400 mg | Phosphorus: 100-150 mg

Oatmeal with Berries and Maple Syrup

This classic breakfast option can be adapted to fit a diabetic and renal diet by using low-sugar toppings and controlling portion sizes.

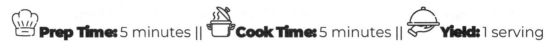 **Prep Time:** 5 minutes || **Cook Time:** 5 minutes || **Yield:** 1 serving

INGREDIENTS

- 1/2 cup rolled oats
- 1 cup water
- Pinch of salt
- 1/4 cup mixed berries (fresh or frozen)
- 1 teaspoon pure maple syrup (optional, use sparingly)
- Cinnamon (optional)

INSTRUCTIONS:

1. Combine oats, water, and salt in a small saucepan.
2. Bring to a boil, then reduce heat and simmer for 5 minutes, or until desired consistency.
3. Remove from heat and stir in mixed berries.
4. Sweeten with a small amount of pure maple syrup, if desired.
5. Sprinkle with cinnamon for added flavor.

NOTES:

- Use old-fashioned oats for a higher fiber content.
- Top with a sprinkle of nuts or seeds for added texture and protein.
- Monitor portion sizes and blood sugar levels carefully.

NUTRITIONAL INFO (approximate per serving):

- Calories: 150-200 | Protein: 5-7 g | Fat: 2-4 g | Carbohydrates: 25-30 g | Sodium: 100-150 mg (may vary based on ingredients) | Potassium: 200-300 mg | Phosphorus: 100-150 mg

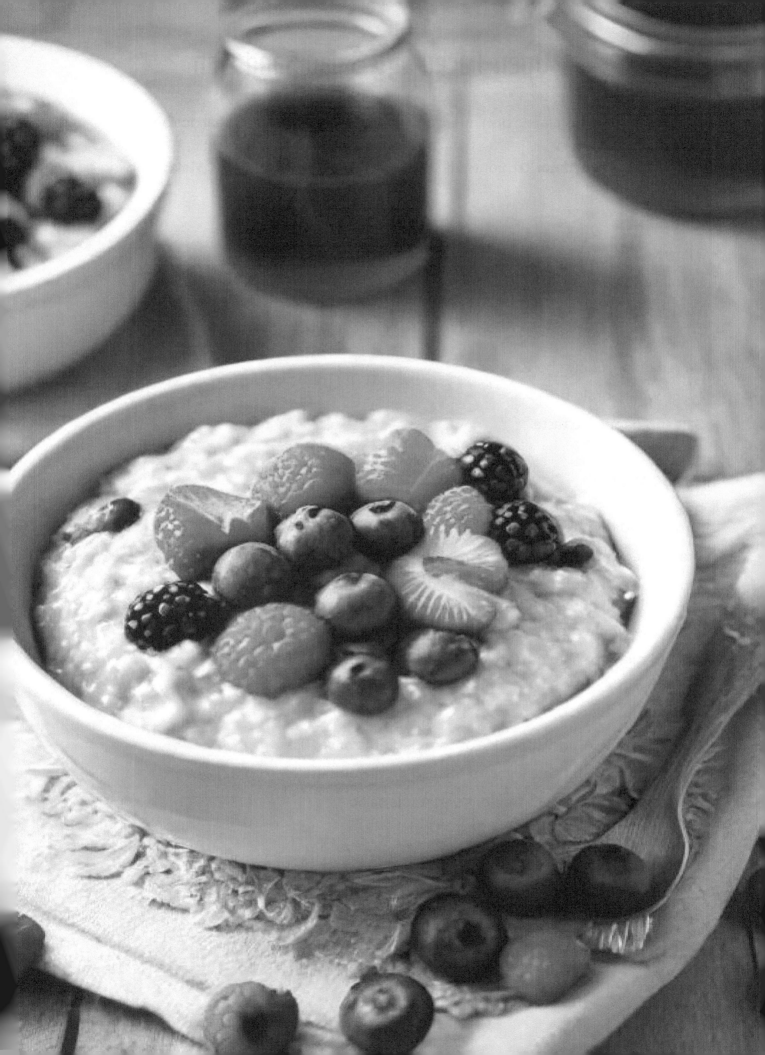

Open-Faced Egg Salad Sandwich

This classic dish offers a light and protein-packed meal option.

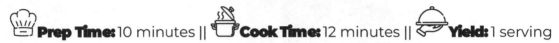 **Prep Time:** 10 minutes || **Cook Time:** 12 minutes || **Yield:** 1 serving

INGREDIENTS

- 2 large eggs

- 1 tablespoon low-fat mayonnaise

- 1 teaspoon Dijon mustard

- 1/4 celery stalk, finely chopped

- 1/4 red onion, finely chopped

- 1 slice whole-grain bread

- Salt and pepper to taste

INSTRUCTIONS:

1. Place eggs in a small saucepan and cover with cold water. Bring to a boil, then reduce heat and simmer for 10 minutes.

2. Transfer eggs to an ice bath to cool rapidly. Peel and chop eggs.

3. In a small bowl, combine chopped eggs, mayonnaise, Dijon mustard, celery, and red onion. Season with salt and pepper.

4. Toast the whole-grain bread.

5. Spread the egg salad mixture generously on the toast.

NOTES:

- For extra protein, add a sprinkle of chopped nuts or seeds.

- You can use low-fat Greek yogurt instead of mayonnaise for a lighter option.

- Serve with a side of fresh fruit or a vegetable salad.

NUTRITIONAL INFO (approximate per serving):

- Calories: 200-250 | Protein: 15-20 g | Fat: 5-8 g | Carbohydrates: 20-25 g | Sodium: 100-150 mg (may vary based on ingredients) | Potassium: 200-300 mg | Phosphorus: 100-150 mg

Breakfast Frittata

This protein-packed frittata is a hearty and satisfying breakfast option.

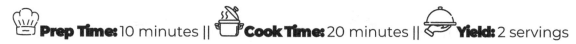 **Prep Time:** 10 minutes || **Cook Time:** 20 minutes || **Yield:** 2 servings

INGREDIENTS

- 4 eggs
- 1/4 cup egg whites
- 1/4 cup reduced-fat cheese (e.g., cheddar, mozzarella)
- 1/2 cup spinach, chopped
- 1/4 cup onion, chopped
- 1/4 cup bell pepper, chopped
- 1/4 teaspoon garlic powder
- Salt and pepper to taste

INSTRUCTIONS:

1. Preheat oven to 375°F (190°C).

2. In a large bowl, whisk together eggs and egg whites. Stir in cheese, spinach, onion, bell pepper, and garlic powder. Season with salt and pepper.

3. Pour mixture into a greased oven-safe skillet or dish.

4. Bake for 18-20 minutes, or until frittata is set and golden brown on top.

NOTES:

- For a lower-carb option, serve with a side of avocado or a handful of berries.
- You can add other vegetables, such as mushrooms or tomatoes, to the frittata.
- Experiment with different types of cheese for added flavor.

NUTRITIONAL INFO (approximate per serving):

- Calories: 250-300 | Protein: 20-25 g | Fat: 10-12 g | Carbohydrates: 5-10 g | Sodium: 100-150 mg (may vary based on ingredients) | Potassium: 200-300 mg | Phosphorus: 100-150 mg

Protein Waffles

These protein-packed waffles are a great way to start your day.

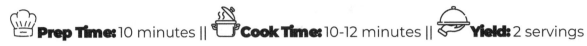 **Prep Time:** 10 minutes || **Cook Time:** 10-12 minutes || **Yield:** 2 servings

INGREDIENTS

- 1/2 cup protein powder (unflavored)
- 2 egg whites
- 1/4 cup unsweetened almond milk
- 1/4 cup whole-wheat flour
- 1 teaspoon baking powder
- 1/4 teaspoon baking soda
- Pinch of salt
- Optional toppings: sugar-free syrup, fresh berries, nuts

INSTRUCTIONS:

1. In a bowl, whisk together protein powder, egg whites, almond milk, whole-wheat flour, baking powder, baking soda, and salt until smooth.

2. Preheat a waffle iron according to manufacturer's instructions.

3. Pour batter onto the preheated waffle iron and cook according to instructions.

4. Serve immediately with desired toppings.

NOTES:

- For a crispier waffle, cook for an extra minute or two.
- Experiment with different flavorings by adding vanilla extract, cocoa powder, or cinnamon to the batter.
- Serve with a side of Greek yogurt for extra protein.

NUTRITIONAL INFO (approximate per serving):

- Calories: 200-250 | Protein: 25-30 g | Fat: 5-8 g | Carbohydrates: 15-20 g | Sodium: 100-150 mg (may vary based on ingredients) | Potassium: 200-300 mg | Phosphorus: 100-150 mg

Protein Pancakes

These pancakes are packed with protein and low in carbohydrates, making them a suitable option for a diabetic and renal diet.

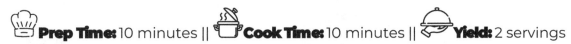

Prep Time: 10 minutes || **Cook Time:** 10 minutes || **Yield:** 2 servings

INGREDIENTS

- 1/2 cup protein powder (unflavored)
- 2 egg whites
- 1/4 cup unsweetened almond milk
- 1 tablespoon whole-wheat flour
- 1 teaspoon baking powder
- Pinch of salt
- Optional toppings: sugar-free syrup, fresh berries, nuts

INSTRUCTIONS:

1. In a bowl, whisk together protein powder, egg whites, almond milk, whole-wheat flour, baking powder, and salt until smooth.

2. Heat a lightly oiled nonstick skillet over medium heat.

3. Pour 1/4 cup of batter onto the skillet for each pancake. Cook until bubbles form on the surface, then flip and cook until golden brown.

4. Serve immediately with desired toppings.

NOTES:

- For a sweeter flavor, use a natural sweetener like stevia or monk fruit extract.
- You can add other flavorings to the batter, such as vanilla extract or cocoa powder.
- Serve with a side of Greek yogurt for extra protein.

NUTRITIONAL INFO (approximate per serving):

- Calories: 150-200 | Protein: 20-25 g | Fat: 2-4 g | Carbohydrates: 10-15 g | Sodium: 100-150 mg (may vary based on ingredients) | Potassium: 200-300 mg | Phosphorus: 100-150 mg

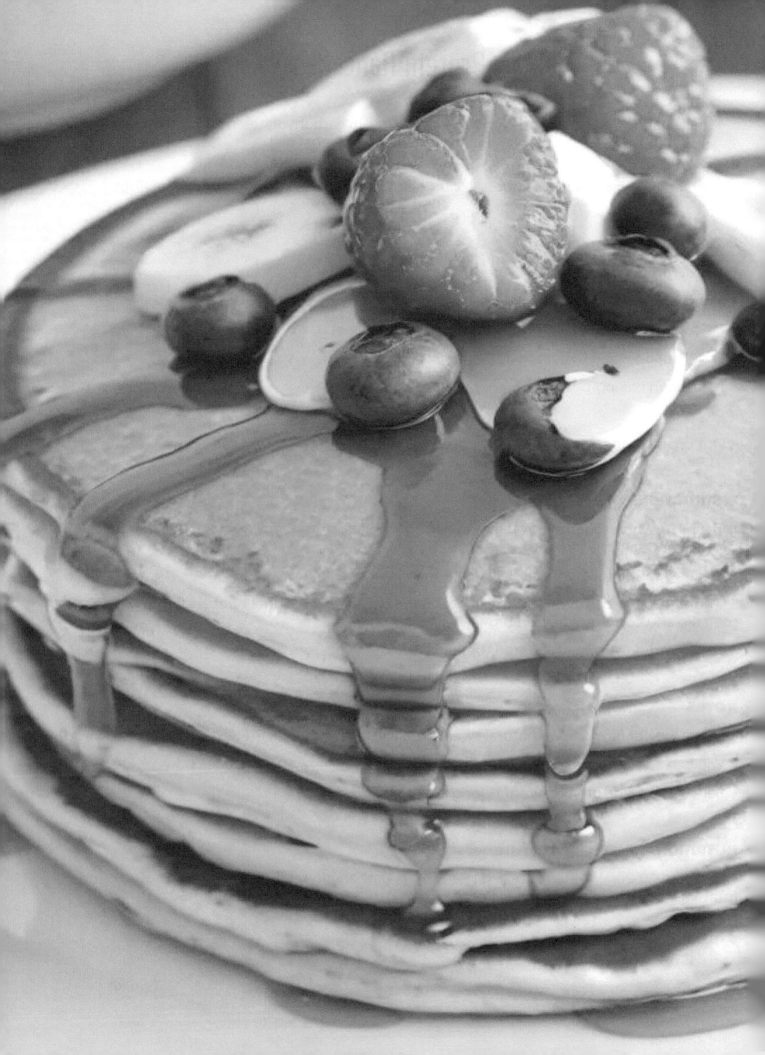

Breakfast Burritos

This recipe offers a satisfying and protein-packed breakfast option.

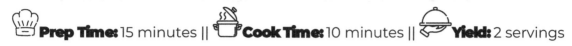 **Prep Time:** 15 minutes || **Cook Time:** 10 minutes || **Yield:** 2 servings

INGREDIENTS

- 2 whole-wheat tortillas
- 2 eggs, scrambled
- 1/2 cup cooked black beans, rinsed and drained
- 1/4 cup diced onion

- 1/4 cup diced green bell pepper
- 1/4 cup shredded low-fat cheddar cheese
- 1/4 avocado, sliced
- Salsa (low-sodium), optional
- Hot sauce, optional

INSTRUCTIONS:

1. Heat a large skillet over medium heat. Scramble eggs and set aside.

2. In the same skillet, sauté onion and green bell pepper until softened.

3. Warm tortillas in a separate pan or microwave.

4. Spread a layer of black beans on each tortilla.

5. Top with scrambled eggs, sautéed vegetables, and shredded cheese.

6. Add avocado, salsa, and hot sauce to taste.

7. Fold tortillas in half to form burritos.

NOTES:

- For a lower-carb option, use lettuce wraps instead of tortillas.
- You can add other vegetables, such as spinach or mushrooms.
- Experiment with different types of cheese or protein sources.

NUTRITIONAL INFO (approximate per serving):

- Calories: 300-350 | Protein: 20-25 g | Fat: 10-12 g | Carbohydrates: 30-35 g | Sodium: 100-150 mg (may vary based on ingredients) | Potassium: 300-400 mg | Phosphorus: 150-200 mg

SEAFOOD DISHES

Baked Salmon with Asparagus

This simple yet flavorful dish is packed with protein and nutrients.

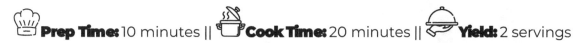 **Prep Time:** 10 minutes || **Cook Time:** 20 minutes || **Yield:** 2 servings

INGREDIENTS

- 2 salmon fillets
- 1 bunch asparagus, trimmed
- 1 tablespoon olive oil
- 1 lemon, sliced
- 1 clove garlic, minced
- Fresh dill, for garnish
- Salt and pepper to taste

INSTRUCTIONS:

1. Preheat oven to 400°F (200°C).

2. In a large baking dish, toss asparagus with olive oil, salt, and pepper.

3. Place salmon fillets on a baking sheet lined with parchment paper.

4. Squeeze lemon juice over salmon and sprinkle with garlic.

5. Roast salmon and asparagus in the preheated oven for 15-20 minutes, or until salmon is cooked through and asparagus is tender.

6. Garnish with fresh dill and lemon slices.

NOTES:

- For added flavor, drizzle salmon with a tablespoon of melted butter before baking.
- You can substitute asparagus with other vegetables like broccoli or green beans.
- Serve with a side of brown rice or quinoa for a complete meal.

NUTRITIONAL INFO (approximate per serving):

- Calories: 250-300 | Protein: 25-30 g | Fat: 10-12 g | Carbohydrates: 5-10 g | Sodium: 100-150 mg (may vary based on ingredients) | Potassium: 200-300 mg | Phosphorus: 100-150 mg

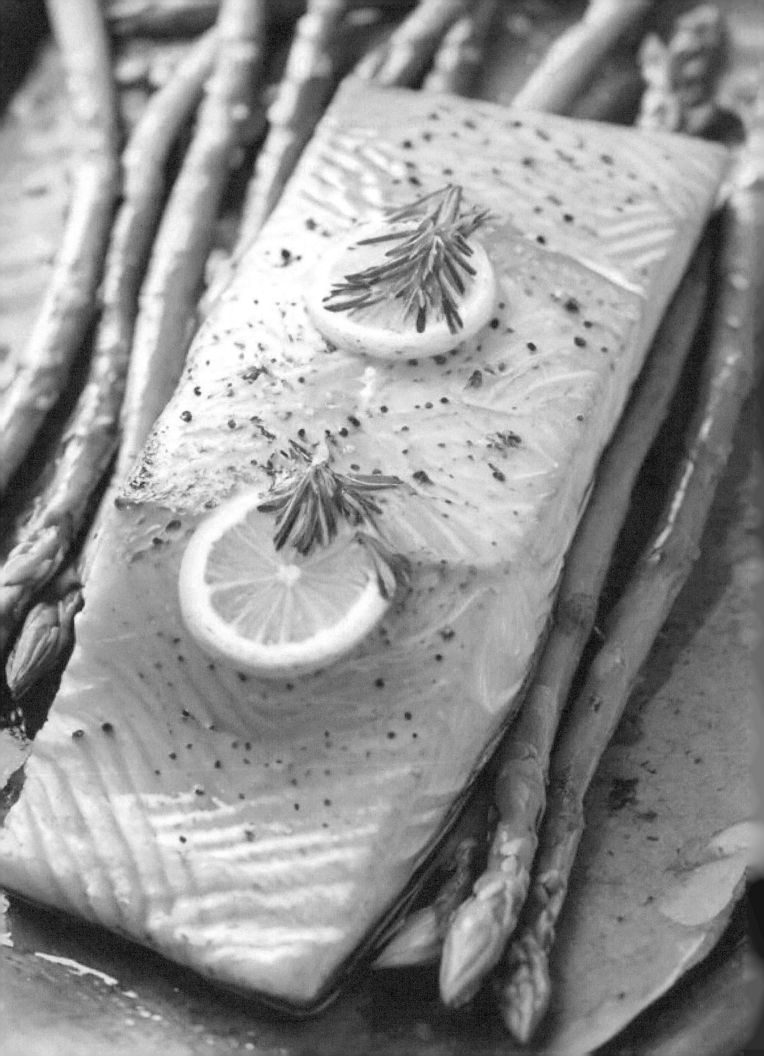

Grilled Shrimp with Zucchini

This dish offers a simple yet flavorful combination of protein and vegetables.

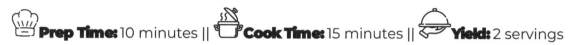 **Prep Time:** 10 minutes || **Cook Time:** 15 minutes || **Yield:** 2 servings

INGREDIENTS

- 1 lb large shrimp, peeled and deveined
- 1 medium zucchini, sliced into thick planks
- 1 tablespoon olive oil
- 1/2 lemon, juiced
- 1/4 teaspoon garlic powder
- 1/4 teaspoon onion powder
- Salt and pepper to taste

INSTRUCTIONS:

1. Preheat your grill to medium-high heat.

2. In a large bowl, combine shrimp, zucchini, olive oil, lemon juice, garlic powder, onion powder, salt, and pepper. Toss to coat.

3. Grill shrimp and zucchini for 5-7 minutes per side, or until shrimp is cooked through and zucchini is tender.

NOTES:

- For extra flavor, marinate the shrimp and zucchini for 15-30 minutes before grilling.
- Serve with a side of brown rice or quinoa for a complete meal.
- You can add other vegetables, such as bell peppers or mushrooms, to the grill.

NUTRITIONAL INFO (approximate per serving):

- Calories: 200-250 | Protein: 25-30 g | Fat: 5-8 g | Carbohydrates: 5-10 g | Sodium: 100-150 mg (may vary based on ingredients) | Potassium: 200-300 mg | Phosphorus: 100-150 mg

Grilled Shrimp with Veggies

This dish is a healthy and flavorful option, perfect for a summer meal.

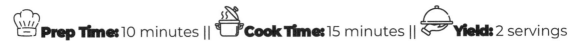 **Prep Time:** 10 minutes || **Cook Time:** 15 minutes || **Yield:** 2 servings

INGREDIENTS

- 1 lb large shrimp, peeled and deveined
- 1 red bell pepper, cut into chunks
- 1 yellow bell pepper, cut into chunks
- 1 zucchini, cut into chunks
- 1 onion, cut into wedges
- 1 tablespoon olive oil
- 1 teaspoon garlic powder
- 1/2 teaspoon onion powder
- 1/4 teaspoon cayenne pepper (optional)
- Salt and pepper to taste

INSTRUCTIONS

1. Preheat your grill to medium-high heat.

2. In a large bowl, combine shrimp, bell peppers, zucchini, onion, olive oil, garlic powder, onion powder, cayenne pepper, salt, and pepper. Toss to coat.

3. Thread the shrimp and vegetables onto skewers.

4. Grill skewers for 5-7 minutes per side, or until shrimp is cooked through and vegetables are tender.

NOTES

- For a lower-carb option, serve with a side salad or cauliflower rice.
- You can adjust the level of spice by adding more or less cayenne pepper.
- Serve with a squeeze of lemon or lime for added flavor.

NUTRITIONAL INFO (approximate per serving):

- Calories: 250-300 | Protein: 25-30 g | Fat: 10-12 g | Carbohydrates: 10-15 g | Sodium: 100-150 mg (may vary based on ingredients) | Potassium: 200-300 mg | Phosphorus: 100-150 mg

Sesame Seared Whitefish

This dish offers a flavorful and crispy crust with the delicate taste of whitefish.

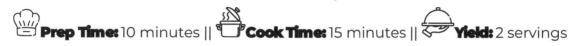 **Prep Time:** 10 minutes || **Cook Time:** 15 minutes || **Yield:** 2 servings

INGREDIENTS

- 2 whitefish fillets
- 1/4 cup sesame seeds
- 1 tablespoon olive oil
- Salt and pepper to taste
- Optional: soy sauce or lime juice for serving

INSTRUCTIONS

1. Preheat a large skillet over medium-high heat.

2. Pat the whitefish fillets dry with paper towels. Season both sides with salt and pepper.

3. In a shallow dish, spread the sesame seeds.

4. Dip each whitefish fillet in the sesame seeds to coat both sides.

5. Add olive oil to the hot skillet. Carefully place the sesame-coated fish fillets in the pan.

6. Cook for 4-5 minutes per side, or until the fish is cooked through and the sesame seeds are golden brown.

7. Remove from the skillet and serve immediately.

NOTES:

- Serve with a side of steamed broccoli or brown rice for a complete meal.
- For extra flavor, squeeze fresh lime juice over the cooked fish.
- You can use a mixture of white and black sesame seeds for added texture.

NUTRITIONAL INFO (approximate per serving):

- Calories: 200-250 | Protein: 25-30 g | Fat: 5-8 g | Carbohydrates: 5-10 g | Sodium: 100-150 mg (may vary based on ingredients) | Potassium: 200-300 mg | Phosphorus: 100-150 mg

Cajun Grilled Whitefish

This recipe delivers a burst of Cajun flavor while keeping the dish light and healthy.

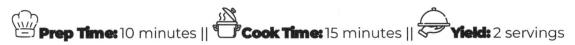 **Prep Time:** 10 minutes || **Cook Time:** 15 minutes || **Yield:** 2 servings

INGREDIENTS

- 2 whitefish fillets (cod, tilapia, or halibut)
- 1 tablespoon Cajun seasoning
- 1/2 teaspoon garlic powder
- 1/4 teaspoon onion powder
- Olive oil spray

INSTRUCTIONS

1. Preheat your grill to medium-high heat.

2. In a small bowl, combine Cajun seasoning, garlic powder, and onion powder.

3. Pat the whitefish fillets dry with paper towels. Generously season both sides with the Cajun spice mixture.

4. Lightly spray the grill grates with olive oil.

5. Place the fish fillets on the preheated grill, skin-side down if applicable.

6. Cook for about 5-7 minutes per side, or until the fish flakes easily with a fork.

7. Remove from grill and serve immediately.

NOTES

- For a low-carb option, serve with a side of steamed broccoli or cauliflower.
- You can adjust the level of spice by adding more or less Cajun seasoning.
- For extra flavor, squeeze fresh lemon juice over the cooked fish.

NUTRITIONAL INFO (approximate per serving):

- Calories: 200-250 | Protein: 25-30 g | Fat: 5-8 g | Carbohydrates: 0 | Sodium: 100-150 mg (may vary based on ingredients) | Potassium: 200-300 mg | Phosphorus: 100-150 mg

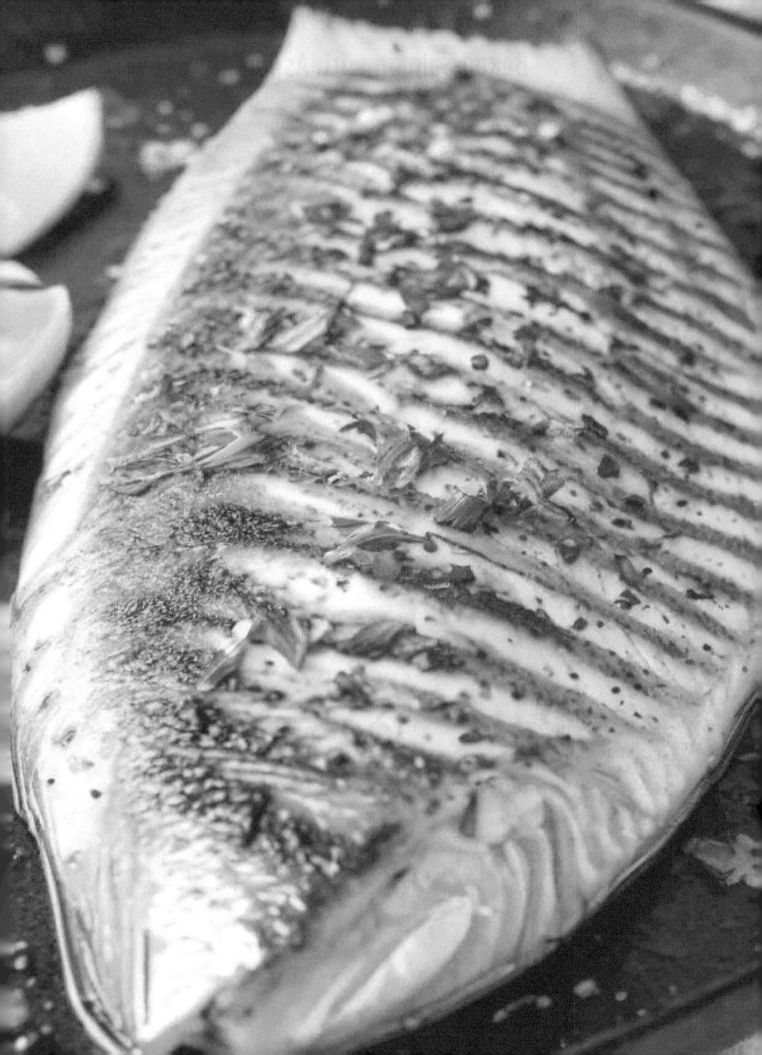

Baked Salmon with Asparagus

This classic combination is a healthy and satisfying meal option.

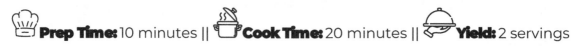 **Prep Time:** 10 minutes || **Cook Time:** 20 minutes || **Yield:** 2 servings

INGREDIENTS

- 2 salmon fillets
- 1 bunch asparagus, trimmed
- 1 tablespoon olive oil
- 1 lemon, sliced
- 1 clove garlic, minced
- Salt and pepper to taste

INSTRUCTIONS:

1. Preheat oven to 400°F (200°C).

2. In a large baking dish, toss asparagus with olive oil, salt, and pepper.

3. Place salmon fillets on a baking sheet lined with parchment paper.

4. Squeeze lemon juice over salmon and sprinkle with garlic.

5. Roast salmon and asparagus in the preheated oven for 15-20 minutes, or until salmon is cooked through and asparagus is tender.

6. Garnish with lemon slices.

NOTES:

- For added flavor, drizzle salmon with a tablespoon of melted butter before baking.
- You can substitute asparagus with other vegetables like broccoli or green beans.
- Serve with a side of brown rice or quinoa for a complete meal.

NUTRITIONAL INFO (approximate per serving):

- Calories: 250-300 | Protein: 25-30 g | Fat: 10-12 g | Carbohydrates: 5-10 g | Sodium: 100-150 mg (may vary based on ingredients) | Potassium: 200-300 mg | Phosphorus: 100-150 mg

Pan-Seared Salmon with Pineapple Salsa

This dish offers a refreshing and flavorful combination of savory salmon and sweet pineapple salsa.

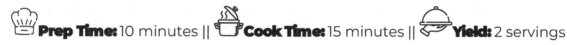 **Prep Time:** 10 minutes || **Cook Time:** 15 minutes || **Yield:** 2 servings

INGREDIENTS

For the Salmon:

- 2 salmon fillets

- 1 tablespoon olive oil

- Salt and pepper to taste

For the Pineapple Salsa:

- 1 cup diced pineapple

- 1/4 cup red onion, finely chopped

- 1/4 cup green bell pepper, finely chopped

- 1 tablespoon fresh lime juice

- 1/2 teaspoon chili powder (optional)

- 1/4 teaspoon cumin (optional)

- Fresh cilantro, chopped, for garnish

INSTRUCTIONS

For the Salmon:

1. Season salmon fillets with salt and pepper.

2. Heat olive oil in a large skillet over medium-high heat.

3. Cook salmon for 4-5 minutes per side, or until cooked through.

For the Pineapple Salsa:

1. In a small bowl, combine pineapple, red onion, green bell pepper, lime juice, chili powder, and cumin.

2. Stir to combine and taste, adjusting seasonings as needed.

To Serve:

- Place cooked salmon on a serving plate.

- Top with pineapple salsa and garnish with fresh cilantro.

NOTES:

- Serve with a side of steamed broccoli or quinoa for a complete meal.

- For a spicier salsa, add a jalapeño or serrano pepper.

- You can adjust the sweetness of the salsa by using less or more pineapple.

NUTRITIONAL INFO (approximate per serving):

- Calories: 250-300 | Protein: 25-30 g | Fat: 10-12 g | Carbohydrates: 10-15 g | Sodium: 100-150 mg (may vary based on ingredients) | Potassium: 200-300 mg | Phosphorus: 100-150 mg

Turmeric Whitefish

This dish offers a flavorful and healthy option, with the added benefits of turmeric.

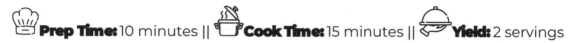 **Prep Time:** 10 minutes || **Cook Time:** 15 minutes || **Yield:** 2 servings

INGREDIENTS

- 4 oz whitefish fillets
- 1 teaspoon ground turmeric
- 1/2 teaspoon garlic powder
- 1/4 teaspoon black pepper
- 1 tablespoon olive oil
- 1 lemon, for squeezing

INSTRUCTIONS

1. Preheat oven to 400°F (200°C).
2. In a small bowl, combine turmeric, garlic powder, and black pepper.
3. Rub the spice mixture evenly over both sides of the whitefish fillets.
4. Heat olive oil in a skillet over medium heat. Briefly sear the fish on both sides for a golden crust.
5. Transfer the fish to a baking sheet lined with parchment paper.
6. Bake for 10-12 minutes, or until the fish flakes easily with a fork.
7. Squeeze fresh lemon juice over the cooked fish.

NOTES

- Serve with a side of roasted vegetables or a green salad for a complete meal.
- You can substitute whitefish with other flaky fish like cod or haddock.
- For added flavor, top with fresh dill or parsley.

NUTRITIONAL INFO (approximate per serving):

- Calories: 200-250 | Protein: 25-30 g | Fat: 5-8 g | Carbohydrates: 5-10 g | Sodium: 100-150 mg (may vary based on ingredients) | Potassium: 200-300 mg | Phosphorus: 100-150 mg

Spicy Shrimp with Veggies

This dish offers a flavorful and healthy option, packed with protein and low in sodium.

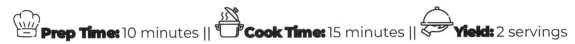 **Prep Time:** 10 minutes || **Cook Time:** 15 minutes || **Yield:** 2 servings

INGREDIENTS

- 8 oz shrimp, peeled and deveined
- 1/2 red bell pepper, sliced
- 1/2 green bell pepper, sliced
- 1/2 onion, sliced
- 1 clove garlic, minced
- 1 tablespoon olive oil

- 1 teaspoon chili powder
- 1/2 teaspoon cumin
- 1/4 teaspoon cayenne pepper (optional)
- 1 tablespoon lime juice
- Salt and pepper to taste

INSTRUCTIONS

1. Pat shrimp dry with paper towels. Season with salt and pepper.

2. Heat olive oil in a large skillet over medium-high heat. Add shrimp and cook until pink and opaque. Remove from skillet and set aside.

3. Add bell peppers and onion to the skillet and cook until softened.

4. Stir in garlic, chili powder, cumin, and cayenne pepper (if using). Cook for 30 seconds, or until fragrant.

5. Return shrimp to the skillet and cook for an additional minute to heat through.

6. Stir in lime juice.

7. Serve immediately over brown rice or quinoa.

NOTES

- For a milder dish, reduce the amount of chili powder and cayenne pepper.
- Serve with a side of avocado or Greek yogurt for a creamy addition.
- You can add other vegetables, such as broccoli or snap peas, to the dish.

NUTRITIONAL INFO (approximate per serving):

- Calories: 250-300 | Protein: 25-30 g | Fat: 10-12 g | Carbohydrates: 10-15 g | Sodium: 100-150 mg (may vary based on ingredients) | Potassium: 200-300 mg | Phosphorus: 100-150 mg

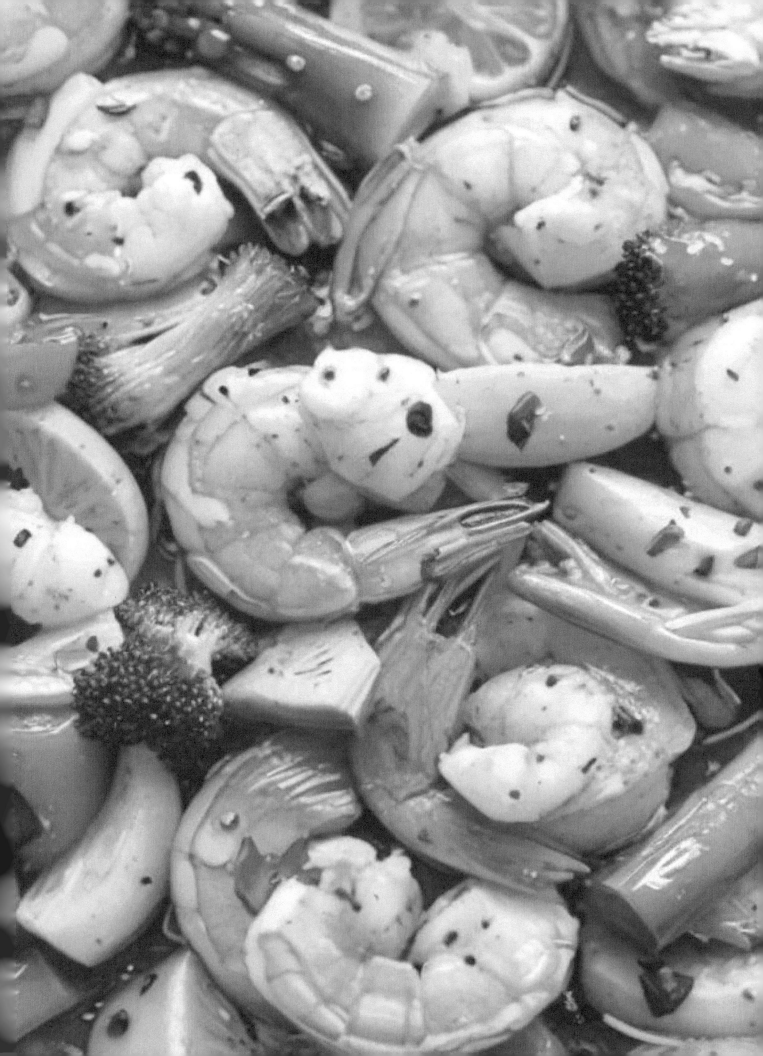

Poached Salmon with Dill Sauce

This delicate dish is a healthy and flavorful option, perfect for a light meal.

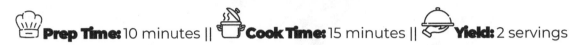 **Prep Time:** 10 minutes || **Cook Time:** 15 minutes || **Yield:** 2 servings

INGREDIENTS

For the Salmon:

- 2 salmon fillets
- 1/2 cup white wine
- 1/2 cup water
- 1 lemon, sliced
- 1 sprig dill
- Salt and pepper to taste

For the Dill Sauce:

- 1/2 cup plain Greek yogurt
- 2 tablespoons fresh dill, chopped
- 1 tablespoon lemon juice
- 1 clove garlic, minced
- Salt and pepper to taste

INSTRUCTIONS

For the Salmon:

1. In a medium saucepan, combine white wine, water, lemon slices, and dill sprig.

2. Season salmon fillets with salt and pepper.

3. Gently place salmon fillets in the poaching liquid.

4. Bring to a simmer over medium heat, then reduce heat to low and cover.

5. Cook for 10-12 minutes, or until salmon is cooked through and flakes easily with a fork.

For the Dill Sauce:

1. In a small bowl, combine Greek yogurt, dill, lemon juice, garlic, salt, and pepper.

2. Stir until well combined.

To Serve:

- Remove salmon from poaching liquid and place on serving plates.
- Top with dill sauce.
- Serve with steamed vegetables or a side salad.

NOTES

- For a richer flavor, add a tablespoon of capers to the dill sauce.

- You can substitute salmon with other white fish, such as cod or haddock.

- Serve with whole-grain bread or crackers, if desired.

NUTRITIONAL INFO (approximate per serving):

- Calories: 200-250 | Protein: 25-30 g | Fat: 5-8 g | Carbohydrates: 5-10 g | Sodium: 100-150 mg (may vary based on ingredients) | Potassium: 200-300 mg | Phosphorus: 100-150 mg

Shrimp Scampi

This classic Italian dish can be adapted to fit a diabetic and renal diet by using low-sodium ingredients and reducing fat.

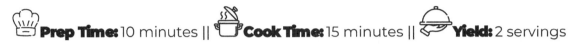 **Prep Time:** 10 minutes || **Cook Time:** 15 minutes || **Yield:** 2 servings

INGREDIENTS

- 8 oz shrimp, peeled and deveined
- 1 tablespoon olive oil
- 1 clove garlic, minced
- 1/4 cup dry white wine (optional)
- 1/4 cup low-sodium chicken broth

- 1 tablespoon lemon juice
- 2 tablespoons capers, drained
- 1/4 teaspoon red pepper flakes (optional)
- 1/4 cup fresh parsley, chopped
- Salt and pepper to taste

INSTRUCTIONS

1. Pat shrimp dry with paper towels. Season with salt and pepper.

2. Heat olive oil in a large skillet over medium-high heat. Add shrimp and cook until pink and opaque. Remove from skillet and set aside.

3. Add garlic to the skillet and cook for 30 seconds, being careful not to burn.

4. Stir in white wine (if using) and chicken broth. Bring to a simmer.

5. Return shrimp to the skillet and add lemon juice, capers, and red pepper flakes. Cook for 1-2 minutes, or until shrimp is heated through.

6. Stir in parsley.

7. Serve immediately with whole-wheat pasta or zucchini noodles.

NOTES

- For a thicker sauce, use a cornstarch slurry.
- Serve with a squeeze of fresh lemon for added flavor.
- You can substitute white wine with additional chicken broth.

NUTRITIONAL INFO (approximate per serving):

- Calories: 200-250 | Protein: 25-30 g | Fat: 5-8 g | Carbohydrates: 5-10 g | Sodium: 100-150 mg (may vary based on ingredients) | Potassium: 200-300 mg | Phosphorus: 100-150 mg

Cod with Lemon and Herbs

This light and flavorful dish is a perfect choice for a quick and healthy meal.

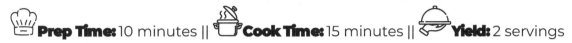 **Prep Time:** 10 minutes || **Cook Time:** 15 minutes || **Yield:** 2 servings

INGREDIENTS

- 8 oz cod fillets

- 1 tablespoon olive oil

- 1 lemon, zested and juiced

- 1 clove garlic, minced

- 1 tablespoon fresh parsley, chopped

- 1 teaspoon dried oregano

- Salt and pepper to taste

INSTRUCTIONS

1. Preheat oven to 400°F (200°C).

2. In a small bowl, combine olive oil, lemon zest, lemon juice, garlic, parsley, oregano, salt, and pepper.

3. Rub the herb mixture over the cod fillets.

4. Place cod on a baking sheet lined with parchment paper.

5. Bake for 15-20 minutes, or until cooked through and flaky.

NOTES

- Serve with a side of roasted vegetables or a green salad for a complete meal.

- You can substitute other white fish for cod, such as haddock or tilapia.

- For a richer flavor, add a dollop of Greek yogurt or sour cream to the fish before serving.

NUTRITIONAL INFO (approximate per serving):

- Calories: 200-250 | Protein: 25-30 g | Fat: 5-8 g | Carbohydrates: 5-10 g | Sodium: 100-150 mg (may vary based on ingredients) | Potassium: 200-300 mg | Phosphorus: 100-150 mg

Seafood Chowder

This light and flavorful chowder is packed with protein and low in sodium, making it a suitable option for a diabetic and renal diet.

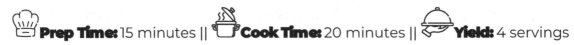 **Prep Time:** 15 minutes || **Cook Time:** 20 minutes || **Yield:** 4 servings

INGREDIENTS

- 1 tablespoon olive oil
- 1 onion, chopped
- 1 celery stalk, chopped
- 1 carrot, diced
- 2 cloves garlic, minced
- 4 cups low-sodium chicken broth
- 1/2 cup low-fat milk
- 1/2 pound cod or haddock, cut into chunks
- 1/4 pound shrimp, peeled and deveined
- 1/4 cup frozen peas
- 1/4 teaspoon dried thyme
- Salt and pepper to taste

INSTRUCTIONS

1. Heat olive oil in a large pot over medium heat. Add onion, celery, and carrot. Cook until softened.

2. Stir in garlic and cook for 30 seconds.

3. Add chicken broth and bring to a boil. Reduce heat and simmer for 10 minutes.

4. Add cod, shrimp, peas, and thyme to the pot. Cook for 5-7 minutes, or until seafood is cooked through.

5. Stir in milk and heat through, but do not boil.

6. Season with salt and pepper to taste.

NOTES

- For a thicker chowder, use a cornstarch slurry.
- You can add other seafood, such as clams or mussels.
- Serve with whole-grain crackers or crusty bread.

NUTRITIONAL INFO (approximate per serving):

- Calories: 200-250 | Protein: 20-25 g | Fat: 5-8 g | Carbohydrates: 10-15 g | Sodium: 100-150 mg (may vary based on ingredients) | Potassium: 200-300 mg | Phosphorus: 100-150 mg

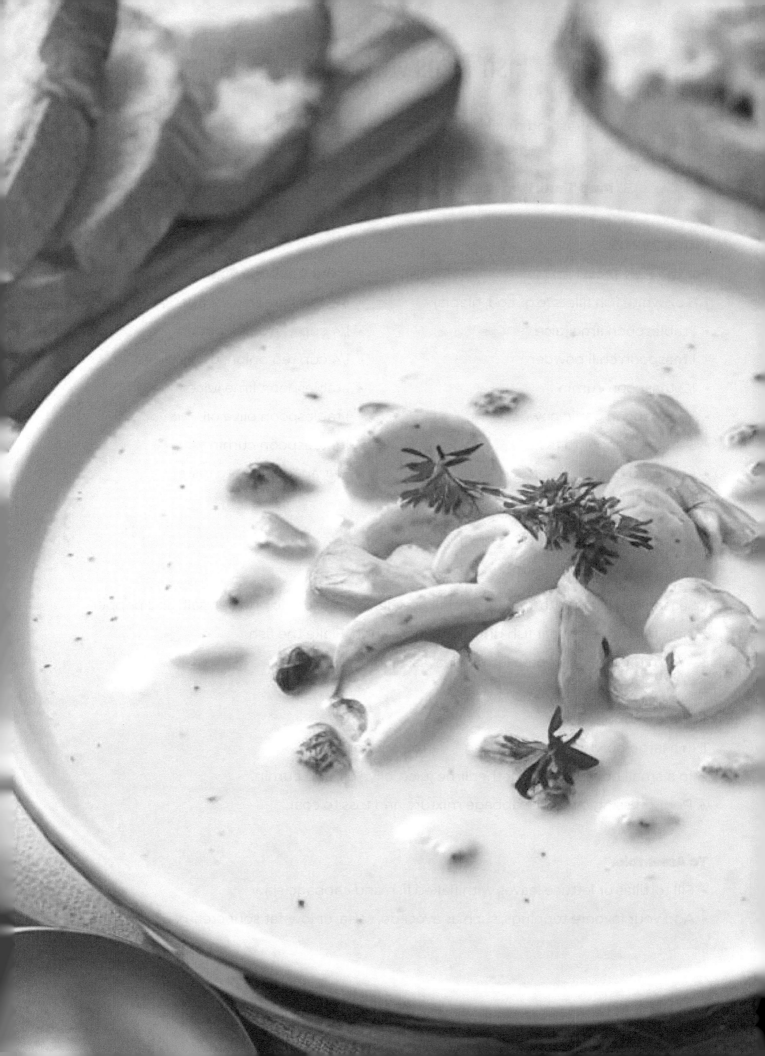

Fish Tacos with Cabbage Slaw

This light and refreshing meal is packed with protein and fiber, making it a perfect option for a diabetic and renal diet.

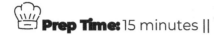 **Prep Time:** 15 minutes || 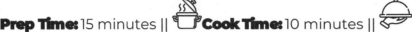 **Cook Time:** 10 minutes || 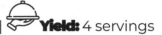 **Yield:** 4 servings

INGREDIENTS

For the Fish Tacos:

- 8 oz white fish fillets (e.g., cod, tilapia)
- 1 tablespoon lime juice
- 1 teaspoon chili powder
- 1/2 teaspoon cumin
- 1/4 teaspoon garlic powder
- Salt and pepper to taste
- Low-carb tortillas or lettuce leaves

For the Cabbage Slaw:

- 1/2 head green cabbage, shredded
- 1/4 cup carrot, shredded
- 1/4 cup red onion, thinly sliced
- 1 tablespoon lime juice
- 1 tablespoon olive oil
- 1/4 teaspoon cumin
- Salt and pepper to taste

INSTRUCTIONS

For the Fish Tacos:

1. Season fish fillets with lime juice, chili powder, cumin, garlic powder, salt, and pepper.

2. Grill, bake, or pan-sear fish until cooked through. Flake the fish.

3. Warm tortillas or prepare lettuce leaves.

For the Cabbage Slaw:

1. In a large bowl, combine cabbage, carrot, and red onion.

2. In a small bowl, whisk together lime juice, olive oil, and cumin.

3. Pour dressing over the cabbage mixture and toss to coat.

To Assemble:

- Fill tortillas or lettuce leaves with flaked fish and cabbage slaw.
- Add your favorite toppings, such as avocado, salsa, or low-fat sour cream.

NOTES

- For a spicier taco, add a pinch of cayenne pepper to the fish seasoning.

- You can adjust the amount of lime juice and cumin to your taste preference.

- Serve with a side of black beans or corn for a more filling meal.

NUTRITIONAL INFO (approximate per serving):

- Calories: 250-300 | Protein: 25-30 g | Fat: 10-12 g | Carbohydrates: 10-15 g | Sodium: 100-150 mg (may vary based on ingredients) | Potassium: 200-300 mg | Phosphorus: 100-150 mg

Shrimp Salad

This light and refreshing salad is packed with protein and healthy fats.

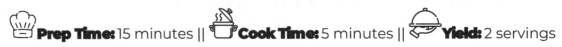 **Prep Time:** 15 minutes || **Cook Time:** 5 minutes || **Yield:** 2 servings

INGREDIENTS

- 8 oz cooked shrimp, peeled and deveined
- 1/4 cup celery, finely chopped
- 1/4 cup onion, finely chopped
- 2 tablespoons low-fat mayonnaise
- 1 tablespoon plain Greek yogurt
- 1 teaspoon Dijon mustard
- 1 tablespoon lemon juice
- 1/4 teaspoon dill
- Salt and pepper to taste

INSTRUCTIONS

1. In a medium bowl, combine shrimp, celery, and onion.

2. In a small bowl, whisk together mayonnaise, Greek yogurt, Dijon mustard, lemon juice, and dill.

3. Add the dressing to the shrimp mixture and stir to combine.

4. Season with salt and pepper to taste.

NOTES

- Serve on a bed of lettuce or with whole-grain crackers.
- You can add other vegetables, such as cucumber or red bell pepper, to the salad.
- For a lower-fat option, use light mayonnaise or Greek yogurt.

NUTRITIONAL INFO (approximate per serving):

- Calories: 200-250 | Protein: 25-30 g | Fat: 5-8 g | Carbohydrates: 5-10 g | Sodium: 100-150 mg (may vary based on ingredients) | Potassium: 200-300 mg | Phosphorus: 100-150 mg

MEAT DISHES

Tarragon Chicken

This dish offers a delicate and flavorful option, perfect for a light and healthy meal.

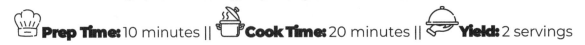 **Prep Time:** 10 minutes || **Cook Time:** 20 minutes || **Yield:** 2 servings

INGREDIENTS

- 4 oz boneless, skinless chicken breast

- 1 tablespoon olive oil

- 1 shallot, finely chopped

- 1/4 cup dry white wine (optional)

- 1/4 cup low-sodium chicken broth

- 2 tablespoons fresh tarragon, chopped

- 1 tablespoon Dijon mustard

- Salt and pepper to taste

INSTRUCTIONS

1. Pat chicken dry with paper towels. Season with salt and pepper.

2. Heat olive oil in a large skillet over medium-high heat. Cook chicken until golden brown and cooked through. Remove from skillet and set aside.

3. Add shallot to the skillet and cook until softened.

4. Stir in white wine (if using) and chicken broth. Bring to a simmer.

5. Return chicken to the skillet and add tarragon and Dijon mustard. Cook for 2-3 minutes, or until chicken is heated through and sauce has thickened slightly.

NOTES

- Serve with a side of steamed broccoli or zucchini for a complete meal.

- You can substitute fresh tarragon with dried tarragon, but use half the amount.

- For a thicker sauce, use a cornstarch slurry.

NUTRITIONAL INFO (approximate per serving):

- Calories: 250-300 | Protein: 25-30 g | Fat: 10-12 g | Carbohydrates: 5-10 g | Sodium: 100-150 mg (may vary based on ingredients) | Potassium: 200-300 mg | Phosphorus: 100-150 mg

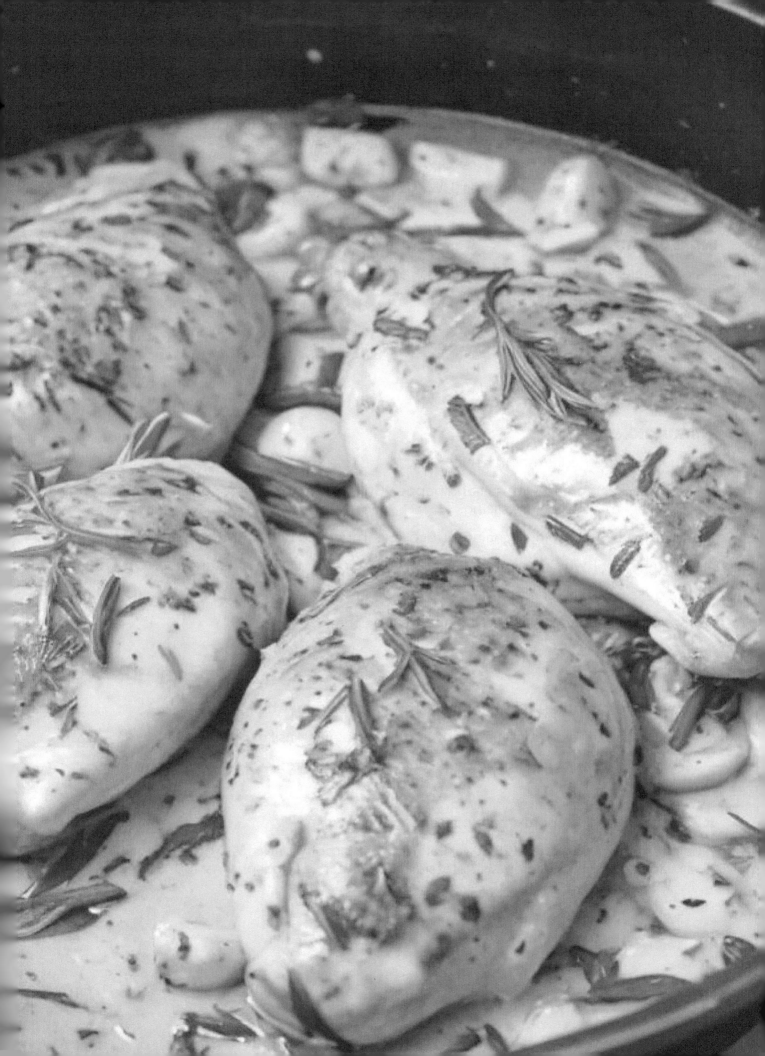

Grilled Chicken Salad

This refreshing salad is packed with protein and nutrients, making it a perfect choice for a light and healthy meal.

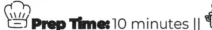 **Prep Time:** 10 minutes || 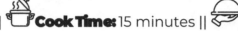 **Cook Time:** 15 minutes || 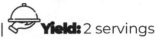 **Yield:** 2 servings

INGREDIENTS

- 4 oz boneless, skinless chicken breast
- 1 head romaine lettuce, chopped
- 1/2 cucumber, sliced
- 1/4 red onion, thinly sliced
- 1/4 cup cherry tomatoes, halved

- 2 tablespoons olive oil
- 1 tablespoon lemon juice
- 1 teaspoon Dijon mustard
- Salt and pepper to taste

INSTRUCTIONS:

1. Preheat grill to medium-high heat.

2. Season chicken breast with salt and pepper. Grill for 8-10 minutes, or until cooked through. Let rest for a few minutes before slicing.

3. In a large bowl, combine romaine lettuce, cucumber, red onion, and cherry tomatoes.

4. In a small bowl, whisk together olive oil, lemon juice, and Dijon mustard.

5. Slice grilled chicken and add to the salad.

6. Drizzle with the prepared dressing and toss to coat.

NOTES:

- For added protein, include a handful of chickpeas or kidney beans.
- You can adjust the dressing flavors by adding herbs like basil or oregano.
- Serve with a side of whole-grain bread or crackers, if desired.

NUTRITIONAL INFO (approximate per serving):

- Calories: 250-300 | Protein: 25-30 g | Fat: 10-12 g | Carbohydrates: 5-10 g | Sodium: 100-150 mg (may vary based on ingredients) | Potassium: 300-400 mg | Phosphorus: 100-150 mg

Baked Chicken with Broccoli

This simple yet satisfying dish is packed with protein and nutrients.

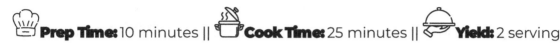 **Prep Time:** 10 minutes || **Cook Time:** 25 minutes || **Yield:** 2 servings

INGREDIENTS

- 4 oz boneless, skinless chicken breast
- 1 head broccoli, cut into florets
- 1 tablespoon olive oil
- 1/2 teaspoon garlic powder
- 1/4 teaspoon onion powder
- Salt and pepper to taste

INSTRUCTIONS

1. Preheat oven to 400°F (200°C).

2. In a large bowl, combine chicken breast, broccoli, olive oil, garlic powder, onion powder, salt, and pepper. Toss to coat evenly.

3. Spread the chicken and broccoli mixture on a baking sheet lined with parchment paper.

4. Bake for 25 minutes, or until chicken is cooked through and broccoli is tender.

NOTES

- For added flavor, squeeze fresh lemon juice over the chicken and broccoli before serving.
- Serve with a side of brown rice or quinoa for a complete meal.
- You can add other vegetables, such as carrots or bell peppers, to the baking sheet.

NUTRITIONAL INFO (approximate per serving):

- Calories: 250-300 | Protein: 25-30 g | Fat: 10-12 g | Carbohydrates: 5-10 g | Sodium: 100-150 mg (may vary based on ingredients) | Potassium: 300-400 mg | Phosphorus: 100-150 mg

Turkey and Avocado Wrap

This light and refreshing wrap is a perfect option for a quick and healthy meal.

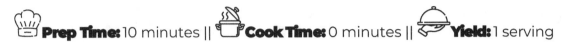

Prep Time: 10 minutes || **Cook Time:** 0 minutes || **Yield:** 1 serving

INGREDIENTS

- 2 oz sliced turkey breast (low-sodium)
- 1/2 avocado, sliced
- 1/4 cup spinach or mixed greens
- 1 tablespoon light mayonnaise or Greek yogurt
- 1/4 tomato, sliced
- 1/4 red onion, thinly sliced
- 1 whole-wheat or low-carb tortilla

INSTRUCTIONS

1. Spread mayonnaise or Greek yogurt on the tortilla.

2. Layer spinach or mixed greens, turkey, avocado, tomato, and red onion on the tortilla.

3. Fold the tortilla in half to create a wrap.

NOTES

- For a lower-carb option, use lettuce leaves instead of a tortilla.
- You can add other vegetables, such as cucumber or bell pepper.
- Experiment with different types of cheese, such as feta or cheddar.

NUTRITIONAL INFO (approximate per serving):

- Calories: 250-300 | Protein: 20-25 g | Fat: 10-12 g | Carbohydrates: 20-25 g | Sodium: 100-150 mg (may vary based on ingredients) | Potassium: 300-400 mg | Phosphorus: 100-150 mg

Turkey Meatballs with Spaghetti Squash

This dish offers a low-carb and protein-packed meal, perfect for those on a diabetic and renal diet.

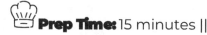 **Prep Time:** 15 minutes || 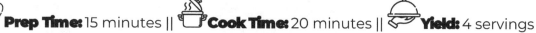 **Cook Time:** 20 minutes || 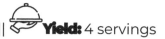 **Yield:** 4 servings

INGREDIENTS

For the Meatballs:

- 1 pound ground turkey

- 1/4 cup bread crumbs (low-sodium)

- 1/4 cup onion, finely chopped

- 1 clove garlic, minced

- 1 egg white

- 1/4 teaspoon dried oregano

- 1/4 teaspoon dried basil

- Salt and pepper to taste

For the Spaghetti Squash:

- 1 medium spaghetti squash

- 1/4 cup marinara sauce (low-sodium)

INSTRUCTIONS

For the Meatballs:

1. Preheat oven to 375°F (190°C).

2. In a large bowl, combine ground turkey, bread crumbs, onion, garlic, egg white, oregano, basil, salt, and pepper.

3. Shape the mixture into meatballs, about 1 inch in diameter.

4. Place meatballs on a baking sheet lined with parchment paper.

5. Bake for 20-25 minutes, or until cooked through.

For the Spaghetti Squash:

1. Cut spaghetti squash in half lengthwise.

2. Scoop out seeds.

3. Place squash face down in a baking dish with a small amount of water.

4. Bake alongside the meatballs for the same amount of time.

5. Once cooked, scrape the flesh with a fork to create spaghetti-like strands.

6. Toss spaghetti squash with marinara sauce.

NOTES

- Serve meatballs with a side of steamed broccoli or green beans for a complete meal.

- You can adjust the seasonings to your taste preference.

- For a richer flavor, add grated Parmesan cheese to the meatballs.

NUTRITIONAL INFO (approximate per serving):

- Calories: 300-350 | Protein: 30-35 g | Fat: 10-12 g | Carbohydrates: 20-25 g | Sodium: 100-150 mg (may vary based on ingredients) | Potassium: 300-400 mg | Phosphorus: 150-200 mg

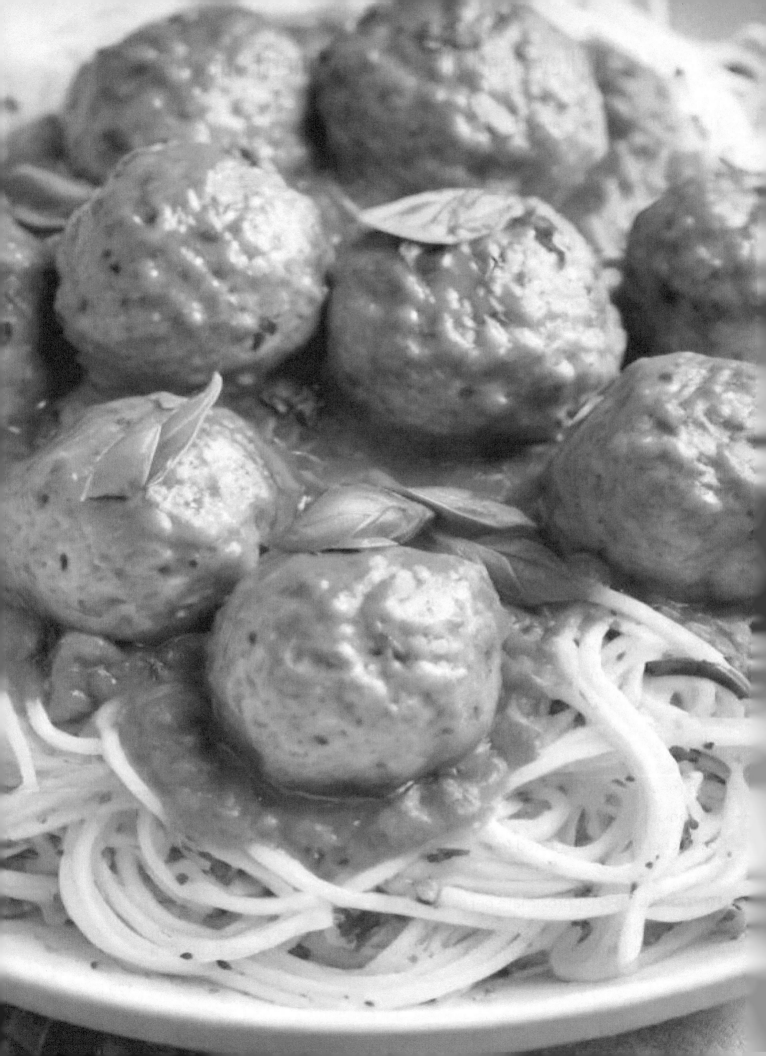

Chicken Satay

This recipe offers a flavorful and satisfying option, with a focus on lean protein and reduced sodium.

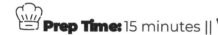**Prep Time:** 15 minutes || 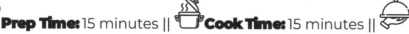**Cook Time:** 15 minutes || 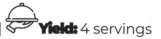**Yield:** 4 servings

INGREDIENTS

For the Chicken:

- 4 oz boneless, skinless chicken breast, thinly sliced

- 1 tablespoon low-sodium soy sauce

- 1 tablespoon lime juice

- 1 clove garlic, minced

- 1/2 teaspoon ground coriander

- 1/4 teaspoon ground cumin

For the Peanut Sauce:

- 1/4 cup natural peanut butter

- 1 tablespoon low-sodium soy sauce

- 1 tablespoon lime juice

- 1 tablespoon rice vinegar

- 1 clove garlic, minced

- 1 tablespoon water (or more, as needed)

INSTRUCTIONS

For the Chicken:

1. In a bowl, combine chicken, soy sauce, lime juice, garlic, coriander, and cumin. Marinate for at least 10 minutes.

2. Grill or pan-sear chicken skewers until cooked through.

For the Peanut Sauce:

1. In a small bowl, combine peanut butter, soy sauce, lime juice, rice vinegar, and garlic.

2. Gradually add water, stirring until desired consistency is reached.

NOTES

- Serve with vegetables like cucumber and carrot sticks for a complete meal.

- You can adjust the spiciness of the peanut sauce by adding a pinch of chili flakes.

- For a lower-carb option, serve with lettuce wraps instead of skewers.

NUTRITIONAL INFO (approximate per serving):

- Calories: 250-300 | Protein: 25-30 g | Fat: 10-12 g | Carbohydrates: 5-10 g | Sodium: 100-150 mg (may vary based on ingredients) | Potassium: 200-300 mg | Phosphorus: 100-150 mg

Pesto Chicken Fettuccine

This recipe offers a flavorful and satisfying meal, combining the creaminess of pesto with the heartiness of chicken.

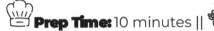 **Prep Time:** 10 minutes || 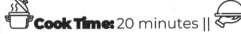 **Cook Time:** 20 minutes || 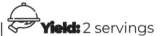 **Yield:** 2 servings

INGREDIENTS

- 4 oz boneless, skinless chicken breast, thinly sliced

- 4 oz whole-wheat fettuccine

- 1/4 cup pesto (low-sodium)

- 1/4 cup low-fat Greek yogurt

- 1/4 cup grated Parmesan cheese (low-sodium)

- 1/4 cup chicken broth

- 1 clove garlic, minced

- 1 tablespoon olive oil

- Salt and pepper to taste

INSTRUCTIONS

1. Cook fettuccine according to package directions. Drain and set aside.

2. Heat olive oil in a large skillet over medium-high heat. Add chicken and cook until browned. Remove from skillet and set aside.

3. In the same skillet, sauté garlic until fragrant.

4. Add pesto, Greek yogurt, Parmesan cheese, and chicken broth to the skillet. Stir until combined and heated through.

5. Return chicken to the skillet and coat with the sauce.

6. Add cooked fettuccine to the skillet and toss to coat evenly.

7. Season with salt and pepper to taste.

NOTES

- For a creamier sauce, use a combination of Greek yogurt and part-skim ricotta cheese.

- You can add other vegetables, such as broccoli or spinach, to the dish.

- Serve with a side salad for a more balanced meal.

NUTRITIONAL INFO (approximate per serving):

- Calories: 400-450 | Protein: 25-30 g | Fat: 15-20 g | Carbohydrates: 40-45 g | Sodium: 100-150 mg (may vary based on ingredients) | Potassium: 200-300 mg | Phosphorus: 150-200 mg

Lemon Artichoke Chicken

This dish offers a light and flavorful option, packed with protein and healthy fats.

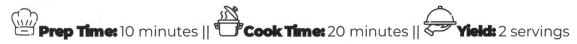 **Prep Time:** 10 minutes || **Cook Time:** 20 minutes || **Yield:** 2 servings

INGREDIENTS

- 4 oz boneless, skinless chicken breast, thinly sliced

- 1 tablespoon olive oil

- 1/2 onion, chopped

- 1 clove garlic, minced

- 1 can (14 ounces) marinated artichoke hearts, drained and chopped

- 1/4 cup low-sodium chicken broth

- 1 tablespoon lemon juice

- 1 teaspoon dried oregano

- Salt and pepper to taste

INSTRUCTIONS

1. Heat olive oil in a large skillet over medium-high heat. Add chicken and cook until browned. Remove from skillet and set aside.

2. Add onion and garlic to the skillet and cook until softened.

3. Stir in artichoke hearts, chicken broth, lemon juice, and oregano. Bring to a simmer.

4. Return chicken to the skillet and cook for a few more minutes, or until chicken is cooked through and sauce has thickened slightly.

5. Season with salt and pepper to taste.

NOTES

- Serve with a side of brown rice or quinoa for a complete meal.

- You can add a squeeze of fresh lemon for extra flavor.

- For a thicker sauce, use a cornstarch slurry.

NUTRITIONAL INFO (approximate per serving):

- Calories: 250-300 | Protein: 25-30 g | Fat: 10-12 g | Carbohydrates: 10-15 g | Sodium: 100-150 mg (may vary based on ingredients) | Potassium: 200-300 mg | Phosphorus: 100-150 mg

Chicken Dumplings

While traditional chicken dumplings might involve rich ingredients, this recipe offers a lighter and healthier alternative suitable for a diabetic and renal diet. We'll focus on a chicken and vegetable soup with dumplings, rather than the traditional meat-filled dumplings.

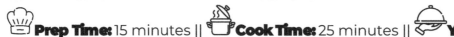 **Prep Time:** 15 minutes || **Cook Time:** 25 minutes || **Yield:** 4 servings

INGREDIENTS

For the Soup:

- 4 cups low-sodium chicken broth

- 1 boneless, skinless chicken breast

- 1 carrot, diced

- 1 celery stalk, diced

- 1/2 onion, chopped

- 1 clove garlic, minced

- 1/2 teaspoon dried thyme

- 1/4 teaspoon black pepper

- Salt to taste

For the Dumplings:

- 1/2 cup all-purpose flour

- 1/4 cup whole-wheat flour

- 1 teaspoon baking powder

- Pinch of salt

- 1/4 cup milk

INSTRUCTIONS

For the Soup:

1. In a large pot, combine chicken broth, chicken breast, carrot, celery, onion, garlic, thyme, and black pepper.

2. Bring to a boil, then reduce heat and simmer for 15 minutes, or until chicken is cooked through.

3. Remove chicken from the soup and shred.

4. Return shredded chicken to the soup.

For the Dumplings:

1. In a small bowl, whisk together flours, baking powder, and salt.

2. Gradually add milk, stirring until a thick batter forms.

3. Drop spoonfuls of batter into the simmering soup.

4. Cook for 5-7 minutes, or until dumplings are cooked through and float to the surface.

NOTES

- For a thicker soup, use a cornstarch slurry.

- You can add other vegetables, such as green peas or corn, to the soup.

- Experiment with different herbs and spices to customize the flavor.

NUTRITIONAL INFO (approximate per serving):

- Calories: 200-250 | Protein: 20-25 g | Fat: 5-8 g | Carbohydrates: 25-30 g | Sodium: 100-150 mg (may vary based on ingredients) | Potassium: 200-300 mg | Phosphorus: 100-150 mg

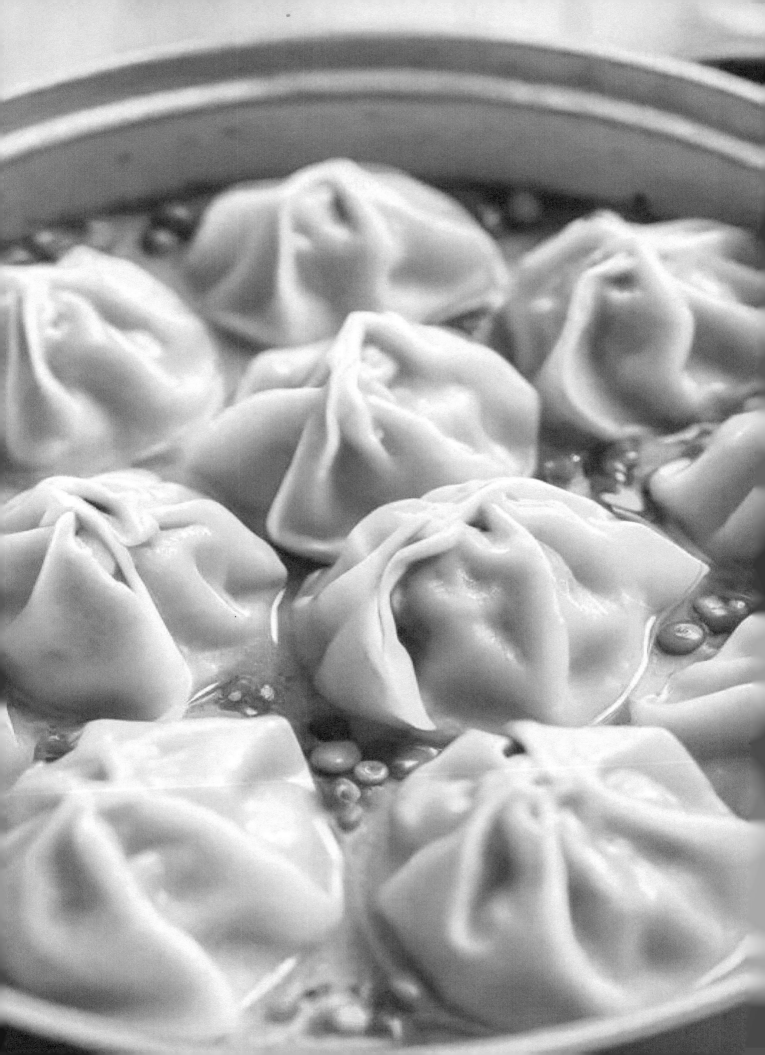

Pesto Chicken

This recipe offers a fresh and flavorful twist on classic chicken.

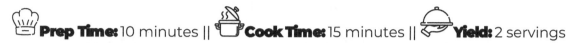 **Prep Time:** 10 minutes || **Cook Time:** 15 minutes || **Yield:** 2 servings

INGREDIENTS

- 4 oz boneless, skinless chicken breast, thinly sliced

- 1 tablespoon olive oil

- 1/4 cup store-bought pesto (low-sodium)

- 1/4 cup grated Parmesan cheese (optional, low-sodium)

- 2 tablespoons chicken broth

- 1 tablespoon lemon juice

- Salt and pepper to taste

- Whole-wheat pasta or zucchini noodles (optional)

INSTRUCTIONS

1. Heat olive oil in a large skillet over medium-high heat. Add chicken and cook until browned. Remove from skillet and set aside.

2. In the same skillet, add pesto and chicken broth. Stir until heated through and sauce is slightly thickened.

3. Return chicken to the skillet and coat with pesto sauce.

4. Stir in lemon juice and Parmesan cheese (if using). Season with salt and pepper.

5. Serve immediately with whole-wheat pasta or zucchini noodles, if desired.

NOTES

- For a homemade pesto, blend fresh basil, pine nuts, garlic, Parmesan cheese, and olive oil in a food processor.

- Serve with roasted vegetables for a complete meal.

- You can adjust the amount of pesto and lemon juice to your taste preference.

NUTRITIONAL INFO (approximate per serving):

- Calories: 250-300 | Protein: 25-30 g | Fat: 10-12 g | Carbohydrates: 10-15 g | Sodium: 100-150 mg (may vary based on ingredients) | Potassium: 200-300 mg | Phosphorus: 100-150 mg

Chicken Fried Rice

This classic dish can be adapted to fit a diabetic and renal diet by using brown rice and low-sodium ingredients.

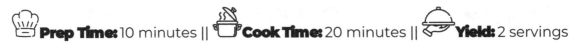 **Prep Time:** 10 minutes || **Cook Time:** 20 minutes || **Yield:** 2 servings

INGREDIENTS

- 4 oz boneless, skinless chicken breast, diced

- 2 cups cooked brown rice

- 1/2 onion, chopped

- 1 carrot, diced

- 1 egg, beaten

- 2 green onions, thinly sliced

- 1 tablespoon soy sauce (low-sodium)

- 1 teaspoon sesame oil

- Salt and pepper to taste

INSTRUCTIONS

1. Heat sesame oil in a large skillet over medium-high heat. Add chicken and cook until browned. Remove from skillet and set aside.

2. Add onion and carrot to the skillet and cook until softened.

3. Push vegetables to the side of the skillet and pour in beaten egg. Scramble until cooked.

4. Stir in cooked rice, chicken, and green onions.

5. Season with soy sauce, salt, and pepper. Cook for a few minutes, or until heated through.

NOTES

- For added flavor, use a mix of frozen peas and corn.

- You can substitute brown rice with cauliflower rice for a lower-carb option.

- Serve with a side of stir-fried vegetables for a more balanced meal.

NUTRITIONAL INFO (approximate per serving):

- Calories: 300-350 | Protein: 25-30 g | Fat: 10-12 g | Carbohydrates: 30-35 g | Sodium: 100-150 mg (may vary based on ingredients) | Potassium: 200-300 mg | Phosphorus: 150-200 mg

Chicken Marsala

This classic Italian dish can be adapted to fit a diabetic and renal diet by using lean chicken and low-sodium ingredients.

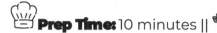 **Prep Time:** 10 minutes || 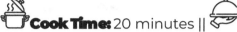 **Cook Time:** 20 minutes || 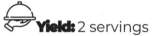 **Yield:** 2 servings

INGREDIENTS

- 4 oz boneless, skinless chicken breast, thinly sliced

- 1/4 cup all-purpose flour

- 1 tablespoon olive oil

- 1/2 cup low-sodium chicken broth

- 1/4 cup Marsala wine (optional, can substitute with extra chicken broth)

- 1 tablespoon capers, drained

- 1/4 cup sliced mushrooms

- 1 clove garlic, minced

- 1 tablespoon fresh parsley, chopped

- Salt and pepper to taste

INSTRUCTIONS

1. Pat chicken dry with paper towels. Season with salt and pepper.

2. Dredge chicken in flour, shaking off excess.

3. Heat olive oil in a large skillet over medium-high heat. Cook chicken until golden brown and cooked through. Remove from skillet and set aside.

4. In the same skillet, sauté garlic and mushrooms until softened.

5. Stir in chicken broth and Marsala wine (if using). Bring to a boil, then reduce heat and simmer for 2-3 minutes, or until sauce thickens slightly.

6. Stir in capers and parsley. Return chicken to the pan and coat with sauce.

7. Serve immediately with a side of whole-wheat pasta or mashed cauliflower.

NOTES

- For a thicker sauce, use a cornstarch slurry.

- Serve with a squeeze of fresh lemon for added flavor.

- You can substitute mushrooms with other vegetables like zucchini or bell peppers.

NUTRITIONAL INFO (approximate per serving):

- Calories: 250-300 | Protein: 25-30 g | Fat: 10-12 g | Carbohydrates: 10-15 g | Sodium: 100-150 mg (may vary based on ingredients) | Potassium: 200-300 mg | Phosphorus: 100-150 mg

Mediterranean Chicken

This dish offers a flavorful and healthy option, packed with Mediterranean flavors.

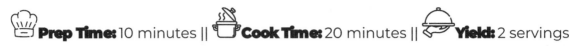 **Prep Time:** 10 minutes || **Cook Time:** 20 minutes || **Yield:** 2 servings

INGREDIENTS

- 4 oz boneless, skinless chicken breast, thinly sliced

- 1 tablespoon olive oil

- 1/2 onion, chopped

- 1 clove garlic, minced

- 1/2 cup cherry tomatoes, halved

- 1/4 cup Kalamata olives, pitted and halved

- 1 tablespoon capers, drained

- 1 teaspoon dried oregano

- 1/2 teaspoon dried basil

- Salt and pepper to taste

- Feta cheese (optional, for serving)

INSTRUCTIONS

1. Heat olive oil in a large skillet over medium-high heat. Add chicken and cook until browned. Remove from skillet and set aside.

2. Add onion and garlic to the skillet and cook until softened.

3. Stir in cherry tomatoes, olives, capers, oregano, and basil. Cook for 2-3 minutes, or until tomatoes start to burst.

4. Return chicken to the skillet and cook for a few more minutes to heat through.

5. Season with salt and pepper to taste.

6. Serve immediately, topped with feta cheese if desired.

NOTES

- Serve with a side of brown rice or quinoa for a complete meal.

- You can add other vegetables, such as zucchini or spinach.

- For a richer flavor, use a splash of white wine while cooking the onions and garlic.

NUTRITIONAL INFO (approximate per serving):

- Calories: 250-300 | Protein: 25-30 g | Fat: 10-12 g | Carbohydrates: 10-15 g | Sodium: 100-150 mg (may vary based on ingredients) | Potassium: 200-300 mg | Phosphorus: 100-150 mg

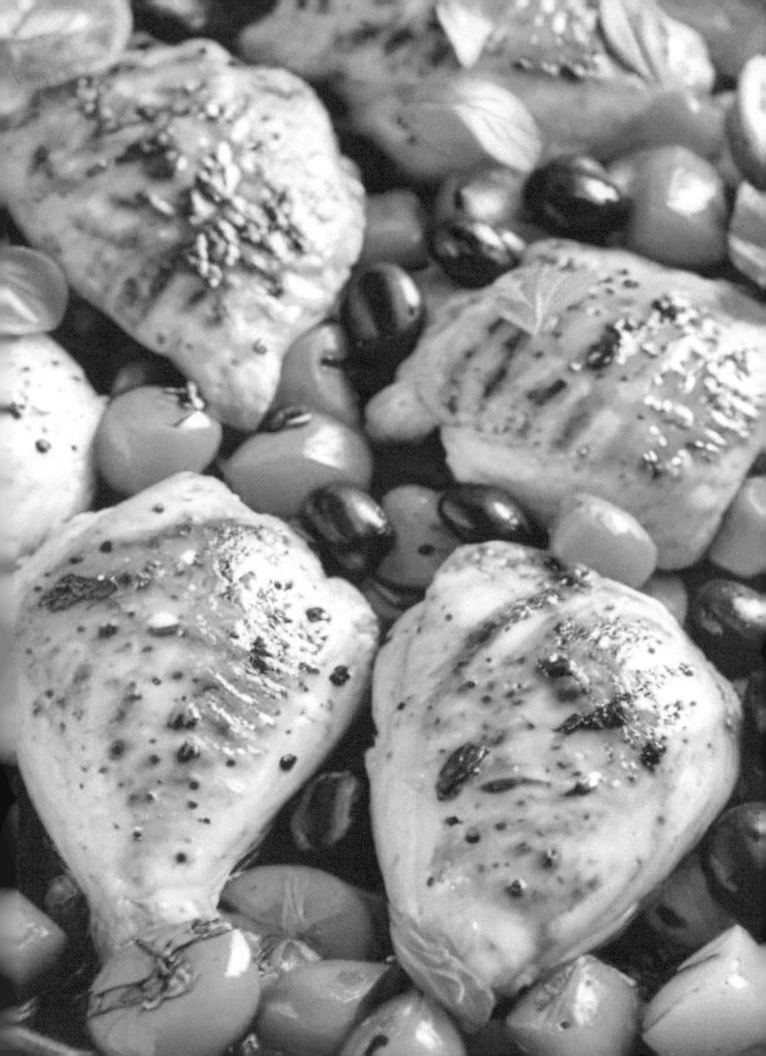

Chicken Fajitas

This dish can be a flavorful and satisfying meal when served with low-carb tortillas or lettuce wraps.

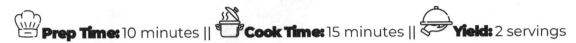 **Prep Time:** 10 minutes || **Cook Time:** 15 minutes || **Yield:** 2 servings

INGREDIENTS

- 4 oz boneless, skinless chicken breast, thinly sliced
- 1 green bell pepper, sliced
- 1 red bell pepper, sliced
- 1 onion, sliced
- 1 clove garlic, minced
- 1 teaspoon chili powder
- 1/2 teaspoon cumin
- 1/4 teaspoon smoked paprika
- 1 tablespoon lime juice
- Low-sodium taco seasoning (optional)
- Low-carb tortillas or lettuce leaves (optional)
- Low-fat sour cream and salsa (optional, for serving)

INSTRUCTIONS

1. Heat a large skillet over medium-high heat with a drizzle of olive oil.

2. Add chicken and cook until browned. Remove from skillet and set aside.

3. Add bell peppers and onion to the skillet and cook until softened.

4. Stir in garlic, chili powder, cumin, and smoked paprika. Cook for 30 seconds, or until fragrant.

5. Return chicken to the skillet and stir to combine.

6. Stir in lime juice and optional taco seasoning.

7. Serve immediately with low-carb tortillas or lettuce leaves. Top with low-fat sour cream and salsa, if desired.

NOTES

- For a vegetarian option, substitute chicken with tofu or firm tempeh.
- Serve with a side of guacamole for added flavor.
- You can adjust the spice level by adding more or less chili powder and smoked paprika.

NUTRITIONAL INFO (approximate per serving):

- Calories: 250-300 | Protein: 25-30 g | Fat: 10-12 g | Carbohydrates: 10-15 g | Sodium: 100-150 mg (may vary based on ingredients) | Potassium: 200-300 mg | Phosphorus: 100-150 mg

Honey Dijon BBQ Chicken

This recipe offers a sweet and tangy flavor profile while being mindful of dietary restrictions.

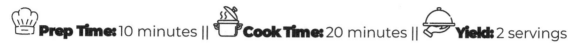 **Prep Time:** 10 minutes || **Cook Time:** 20 minutes || **Yield:** 2 servings

INGREDIENTS

- 4 oz boneless, skinless chicken breast
- 1 tablespoon Dijon mustard
- 1 tablespoon honey
- 1/4 cup low-sodium soy sauce
- 1 clove garlic, minced
- 1/4 teaspoon smoked paprika
- 1/8 teaspoon cayenne pepper (optional)

INSTRUCTIONS

1. Preheat oven to 400°F (200°C).

2. In a small bowl, whisk together Dijon mustard, honey, soy sauce, garlic, smoked paprika, and cayenne pepper.

3. Place chicken breasts in a baking dish and pour the marinade over them, ensuring the chicken is fully coated.

4. Bake for 20-25 minutes, or until chicken is cooked through and the sauce has thickened.

NOTES

- For a quicker option, grill or pan-sear the chicken.
- Serve with a side of steamed broccoli or roasted sweet potatoes.
- You can adjust the sweetness or spiciness by adding more or less honey or cayenne pepper.

NUTRITIONAL INFO (approximate per serving):

- Calories: 250-300 | Protein: 25-30 g | Fat: 5-8 g | Carbohydrates: 10-15 g | Sodium: 100-150 mg (may vary based on ingredients) | Potassium: 200-300 mg | Phosphorus: 100-150 mg

Herb-Roasted Chicken Breast

This recipe offers a flavorful and healthy way to enjoy chicken breast.

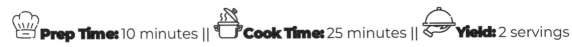 **Prep Time:** 10 minutes || **Cook Time:** 25 minutes || **Yield:** 2 servings

INGREDIENTS

- 4 oz boneless, skinless chicken breast
- 1 tablespoon olive oil
- 1 teaspoon dried rosemary
- 1 teaspoon dried thyme
- 1/2 teaspoon garlic powder
- Salt and pepper to taste

INSTRUCTIONS

1. Preheat oven to 400°F (200°C).

2. In a small bowl, combine olive oil, rosemary, thyme, garlic powder, salt, and pepper.

3. Rub the herb mixture over the chicken breast.

4. Place the chicken on a baking sheet lined with parchment paper.

5. Roast in the preheated oven for 20-25 minutes, or until cooked through.

NOTES

- For added flavor, stuff the chicken breast with lemon slices or fresh herbs.
- Serve with roasted vegetables or a side salad for a complete meal.
- You can adjust the herbs used based on your preference.

NUTRITIONAL INFO (approximate per serving):

- Calories: 150-200 | Protein: 25-30 g | Fat: 5-8 g | Carbohydrates: 0 | Sodium: 100-150 mg (may vary based on ingredients) | Potassium: 200-300 mg | Phosphorus: 100-150 mg

Sour Cream Chicken with Salsa

This dish is a quick and flavorful option, combining the tanginess of salsa with the creaminess of sour cream.

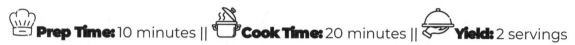 **Prep Time:** 10 minutes || **Cook Time:** 20 minutes || **Yield:** 2 servings

INGREDIENTS

- 4 oz boneless, skinless chicken breast, thinly sliced
- 1 tablespoon olive oil
- 1/2 onion, chopped
- 1 clove garlic, minced
- 1/2 cup salsa (low-sodium)

- 1/4 cup low-fat sour cream
- 1/4 cup low-sodium chicken broth
- 1/4 teaspoon chili powder
- 1/4 teaspoon cumin
- Salt and pepper to taste
- Optional: Tortilla chips or whole-grain bread

INSTRUCTIONS

1. Heat olive oil in a large skillet over medium-high heat. Add chicken and cook until browned. Remove from skillet and set aside.

2. Add onion and garlic to the skillet and cook until softened.

3. Stir in salsa, sour cream, chicken broth, chili powder, and cumin. Bring to a simmer.

4. Return chicken to the skillet and cook until heated through.

5. Season with salt and pepper to taste.

NOTES

- Serve with a side of brown rice or quinoa for a complete meal.
- For a thicker sauce, use a cornstarch slurry.
- You can adjust the spiciness by using a milder or hotter salsa.

NUTRITIONAL INFO (approximate per serving):

- Calories: 250-300 | Protein: 25-30 g | Fat: 10-12 g | Carbohydrates: 10-15 g | Sodium: 100-150 mg (may vary based on ingredients) | Potassium: 200-300 mg | Phosphorus: 100-150 mg

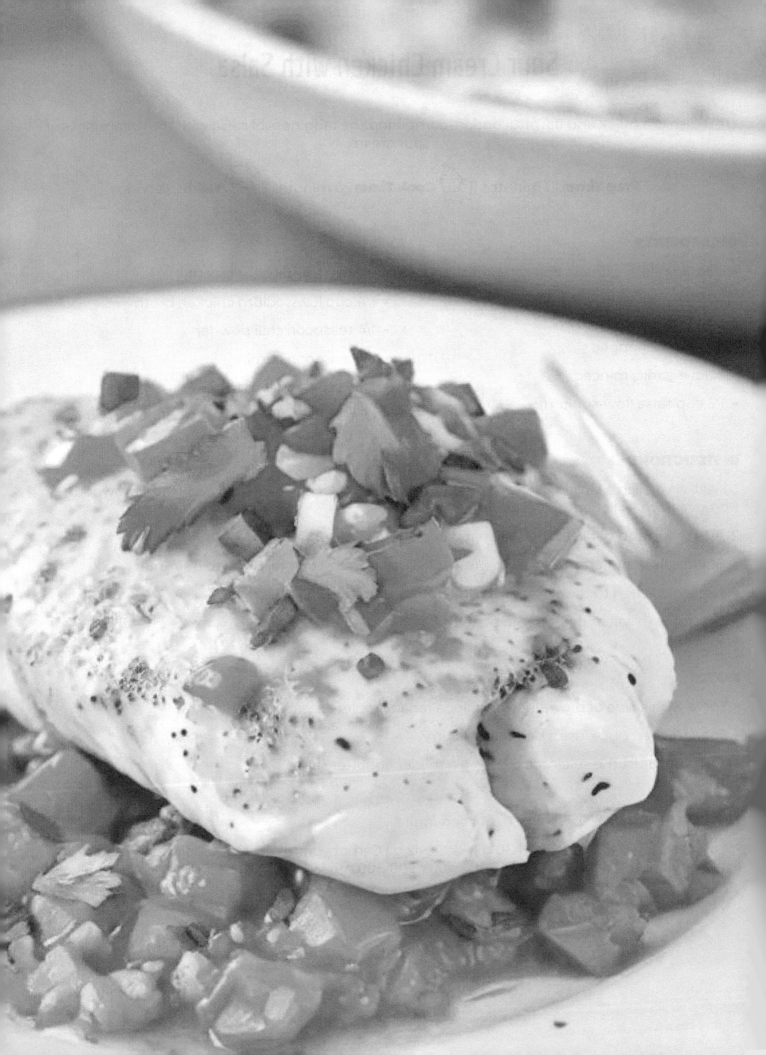

Chicken Piccata

This classic Italian dish can be adapted to fit a diabetic and renal diet by using lean chicken and low-sodium ingredients.

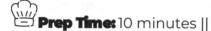**Prep Time:** 10 minutes || 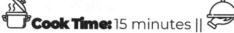**Cook Time:** 15 minutes || 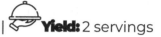**Yield:** 2 servings

INGREDIENTS

- 4 oz boneless, skinless chicken breast, thinly sliced

- 1/4 cup all-purpose flour

- 1 tablespoon olive oil

- 1/2 cup low-sodium chicken broth

- 2 tablespoons lemon juice

- 1 tablespoon capers, drained

- 2 tablespoons fresh parsley, chopped

- Salt and pepper to taste

INSTRUCTIONS

1. Pat chicken dry with paper towels. Season with salt and pepper.

2. Dredge chicken in flour, shaking off excess.

3. Heat olive oil in a large skillet over medium-high heat. Cook chicken until golden brown and cooked through. Remove from skillet and set aside.

4. In the same skillet, add chicken broth and lemon juice. Bring to a boil, then reduce heat and simmer for 2-3 minutes, or until sauce thickens slightly.

5. Stir in capers and parsley.

6. Return chicken to the pan and coat with sauce.

7. Serve immediately with a side of whole-wheat pasta or mashed cauliflower.

NOTES

- For a thicker sauce, use a cornstarch slurry.

- Serve with a squeeze of fresh lemon for added flavor.

- You can substitute lemon juice with white wine for a more traditional flavor.

NUTRITIONAL INFO (approximate per serving):

- Calories: 250-300 | Protein: 25-30 g | Fat: 10-12 g | Carbohydrates: 10-15 g | Sodium: 100-150 mg (may vary based on ingredients) | Potassium: 200-300 mg | Phosphorus: 100-150 mg

Chicken and Farfalle

This dish offers a balance of protein and carbohydrates, making it a satisfying meal option.

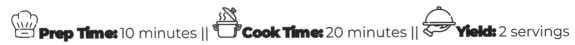 **Prep Time:** 10 minutes || **Cook Time:** 20 minutes || **Yield:** 2 servings

INGREDIENTS

- 4 oz boneless, skinless chicken breast, cut into strips
- 4 oz farfalle pasta
- 1/2 cup broccoli florets
- 1/4 cup red bell pepper, sliced
- 1 clove garlic, minced
- 1/4 cup low-sodium chicken broth
- 1 tablespoon olive oil
- 1 teaspoon dried oregano
- Salt and pepper to taste
- Parmesan cheese (optional)

INSTRUCTIONS

1. Cook farfalle pasta. Drain and set aside.

2. In a large skillet, heat olive oil over medium-high heat. Add chicken and cook until browned. Remove from skillet and set aside.

3. Add broccoli and red bell pepper to the skillet and cook for 2-3 minutes, or until slightly softened.

4. Stir in garlic and cook for 30 seconds.

5. Return chicken to the skillet and pour in chicken broth. Bring to a simmer.

6. Add cooked farfalle to the skillet and toss to coat.

7. Season with oregano, salt, and pepper.

8. Serve immediately, topped with Parmesan cheese if desired.

NOTES

- For a creamier sauce, stir in a tablespoon of low-fat Greek yogurt before serving.
- You can substitute other vegetables, such as spinach or zucchini.
- Use whole-wheat farfalle for a higher fiber option.

NUTRITIONAL INFO (approximate per serving):

- Calories: 300-350 | Protein: 25-30 g | Fat: 10-12 g | Carbohydrates: 30-35 g | Sodium: 100-150 mg (may vary based on ingredients) | Potassium: 300-400 mg | Phosphorus: 150-200 mg

Honey Garlic Chicken

This flavorful dish is a great source of protein and can be a satisfying meal when paired with a side of vegetables.

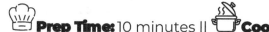 **Prep Time:** 10 minutes || 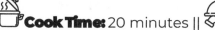 **Cook Time:** 20 minutes || 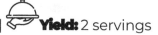 **Yield:** 2 servings

INGREDIENTS

- 4 oz boneless, skinless chicken breast, thinly sliced

- 1 tablespoon olive oil

- 2 cloves garlic, minced

- 1 tablespoon low-sodium soy sauce

- 1 tablespoon honey

- 1 teaspoon rice vinegar

- 1/4 teaspoon red pepper flakes (optional)

- 1 tablespoon cornstarch

- 1 tablespoon water

INSTRUCTIONS

1. In a small bowl, whisk together soy sauce, honey, rice vinegar, red pepper flakes, cornstarch, and water. Set aside.

2. Heat olive oil in a large skillet over medium-high heat. Add chicken and cook until browned.

3. Add garlic to the skillet and cook for 30 seconds.

4. Pour the sauce over the chicken and bring to a boil. Reduce heat and simmer until sauce thickens.

5. Serve immediately with a side of brown rice or quinoa.

NOTES

- For a thicker sauce, use additional cornstarch.

- Serve with steamed broccoli or green beans for a balanced meal.

- Adjust the amount of red pepper flakes to your taste preference.

NUTRITIONAL INFO (approximate per serving):

- Calories: 250-300 | Protein: 25-30 g | Fat: 10-12 g | Carbohydrates: 10-15 g | Sodium: 100-150 mg (may vary based on ingredients) | Potassium: 200-300 mg | Phosphorus: 100-150 mg

Chicken Salad Sandwiches

This light and refreshing sandwich is a great option for a quick and healthy lunch.

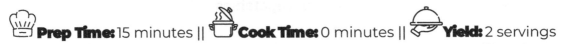 **Prep Time:** 15 minutes || **Cook Time:** 0 minutes || **Yield:** 2 servings

INGREDIENTS

- 4 oz cooked chicken breast, shredded
- 1/4 cup celery, chopped
- 1/4 cup onion, chopped
- 2 tablespoons low-fat mayonnaise
- 1 tablespoon plain Greek yogurt
- 1 teaspoon Dijon mustard
- Salt and pepper to taste
- 4 slices whole-grain bread

INSTRUCTIONS

1. In a medium bowl, combine shredded chicken, celery, and onion.

2. In a small bowl, whisk together mayonnaise, Greek yogurt, and Dijon mustard.

3. Add the dressing to the chicken mixture and stir to combine.

4. Season with salt and pepper to taste.

5. Spread the chicken salad mixture on four slices of whole-grain bread.

NOTES

- For a lower-carb option, use lettuce wraps instead of bread.
- You can add other vegetables to the salad, such as carrots or grapes.
- Experiment with different types of mustard for added flavor.

NUTRITIONAL INFO (approximate per serving):

- Calories: 250-300 | Protein: 25-30 g | Fat: 10-12 g | Carbohydrates: 25-30 g | Sodium: 100-150 mg (may vary based on ingredients) | Potassium: 300-400 mg | Phosphorus: 150-200 mg

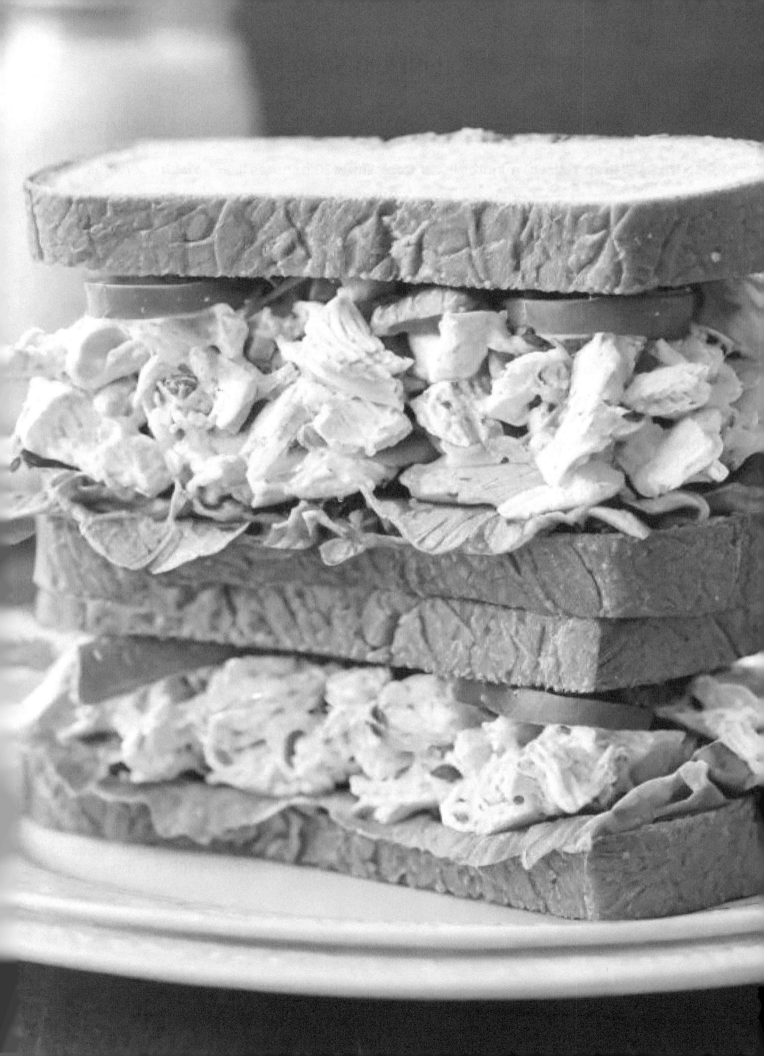

Chicken Soup

This comforting and nourishing soup is a great option for a quick and healthy meal.

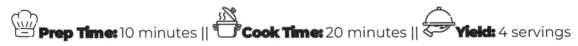 **Prep Time:** 10 minutes || **Cook Time:** 20 minutes || **Yield:** 4 servings

INGREDIENTS

- 1 boneless, skinless chicken breast
- 4 cups low-sodium chicken broth
- 1 carrot, diced
- 1 celery stalk, diced
- 1/2 onion, chopped

- 1 clove garlic, minced
- 1/4 teaspoon dried thyme
- 1/4 teaspoon black pepper
- Salt to taste
- Egg noodles (optional)

INSTRUCTIONS

1. In a medium saucepan, combine chicken, chicken broth, carrot, celery, onion, garlic, thyme, and black pepper.

2. Bring to a boil, then reduce heat and simmer for 15-20 minutes, or until chicken is cooked through.

3. Remove chicken from the soup and shred.

4. Return shredded chicken to the soup.

5. If desired, cook egg noodles and add to soup.

6. Season with salt to taste.

NOTES

- For a thicker soup, use a cornstarch slurry.
- You can add other vegetables, such as spinach or kale, to the soup.
- Serve with crusty bread or a side salad.

NUTRITIONAL INFO (approximate per serving):

- Calories: 150-200 | Protein: 20-25 g | Fat: 2-4 g | Carbohydrates: 10-15 g | Sodium: 100-150 mg (may vary based on ingredients) | Potassium: 200-300 mg | Phosphorus: 100-150 mg

Chicken Breast and Veggie Kebabs

This dish is a healthy and satisfying option, packed with protein and fiber. The grilling method helps to reduce fat content.

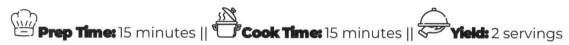 **Prep Time:** 15 minutes || **Cook Time:** 15 minutes || **Yield:** 2 servings

INGREDIENTS

- 4 oz boneless, skinless chicken breast, cut into cubes
- 1 red bell pepper, cut into chunks
- 1 green bell pepper, cut into chunks
- 1 yellow onion, cut into chunks
- 1 tablespoon olive oil
- 1 teaspoon dried oregano
- 1/2 teaspoon garlic powder
- Salt and pepper to taste

INSTRUCTIONS

1. In a bowl, combine chicken, bell peppers, onion, olive oil, oregano, garlic powder, salt, and pepper. Toss to coat evenly.

2. Soak metal skewers in water for 15 minutes to prevent sticking.

3. Thread chicken and vegetables alternately onto skewers.

4. Preheat grill to medium-high heat.

5. Grill kebabs for 10-12 minutes, or until chicken is cooked through and vegetables are tender, turning occasionally.

NOTES

- For a quicker option, use pre-cut vegetables.
- Serve with a side of brown rice or quinoa for a complete meal.
- You can adjust the seasonings to your taste preference.

NUTRITIONAL INFO (approximate per serving):

- Calories: 250-300 | Protein: 25-30 g | Fat: 10-12 g | Carbohydrates: 10-15 g | Sodium: 100-150 mg (may vary based on ingredients) | Potassium: 300-400 mg | Phosphorus: 150-200 mg

Chicken and Vegetable Curry

This light and flavorful curry is packed with protein and fiber, making it a healthy option for individuals with diabetes and kidney disease.

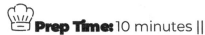 **Prep Time:** 10 minutes || 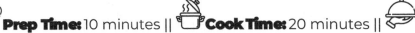 **Cook Time:** 20 minutes || 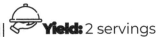 **Yield:** 2 servings

INGREDIENTS

- 4 oz boneless, skinless chicken breast, cut into bite-sized pieces
- 1 onion, chopped
- 1 green bell pepper, sliced
- 1 carrot, diced
- 1 clove garlic, minced
- 1 teaspoon ground cumin
- 1 teaspoon ground coriander
- 1/2 teaspoon turmeric
- 1/4 teaspoon cayenne pepper (optional)
- 1 can (15 ounces) light coconut milk
- 1 cup low-sodium chicken broth
- Fresh cilantro, for garnish

INSTRUCTIONS

1. Heat a large skillet over medium heat with a drizzle of olive oil.

2. Add chicken and cook until browned. Remove from skillet and set aside.

3. Add onion, green pepper, carrot, and garlic to the skillet. Sauté until softened.

4. Stir in cumin, coriander, turmeric, and cayenne pepper. Cook for 30 seconds, or until fragrant.

5. Return chicken to the skillet. Pour in coconut milk and chicken broth. Bring to a simmer.

6. Reduce heat and let simmer for 15 minutes, or until chicken is cooked through and sauce has thickened. Garnish with fresh cilantro before serving.

NOTES

- Serve with brown rice or cauliflower rice for a complete meal.
- You can adjust the level of spice by adding more or less cayenne pepper.
- For a thicker curry, use a cornstarch slurry.
- To reduce sodium content, use fresh garlic and ginger instead of pre-minced or powdered varieties.

NUTRITIONAL INFO (approximate per serving):

- Calories: 250-300 | Protein: 25-30 g | Fat: 10-12 g | Carbohydrates: 15-20 g | Sodium: 100-150 mg (may vary based on ingredients) | Potassium: 300-400 mg | Phosphorus: 150-200 mg

Beef Stir-Fry with Peppers

This quick and flavorful stir-fry is a great option for a busy weeknight. The combination of lean beef and colorful peppers provides a nutritious and satisfying meal.

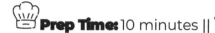**Prep Time:** 10 minutes || 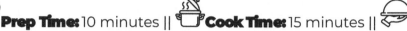**Cook Time:** 15 minutes || 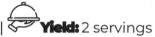**Yield:** 2 servings

INGREDIENTS

- 8 oz lean flank steak, thinly sliced
- 1 red bell pepper, sliced
- 1 green bell pepper, sliced
- 1 onion, sliced
- 2 cloves garlic, minced

- 1 tablespoon low-sodium soy sauce
- 1 tablespoon rice vinegar
- 1 teaspoon cornstarch
- 1/4 teaspoon red pepper flakes (optional)
- 1 teaspoon sesame oil

INSTRUCTIONS

1. In a small bowl, whisk together soy sauce, rice vinegar, cornstarch, and red pepper flakes. Set aside.

2. Heat sesame oil in a large skillet or wok over high heat.

3. Add beef and stir-fry until browned. Remove from skillet and set aside.

4. Add onion and peppers to the skillet and stir-fry until softened.

5. Return beef to the skillet and pour the sauce over the mixture. Bring to a boil, then reduce heat and simmer until sauce thickens.

6. Serve immediately over brown rice or cauliflower rice.

NOTES

- For a lower-carb option, serve over zucchini noodles or shirataki noodles.
- You can add other vegetables to the stir-fry, such as broccoli or snow peas.
- Adjust the amount of red pepper flakes to your taste preference.

NUTRITIONAL INFO (approximate per serving):

- Calories: 250-300 | Protein: 25-30 g | Fat: 10-12 g | Carbohydrates: 10-15 g | Sodium: 100-150 mg (may vary based on ingredients) | Potassium: 200-300 mg | Phosphorus: 100-150 mg

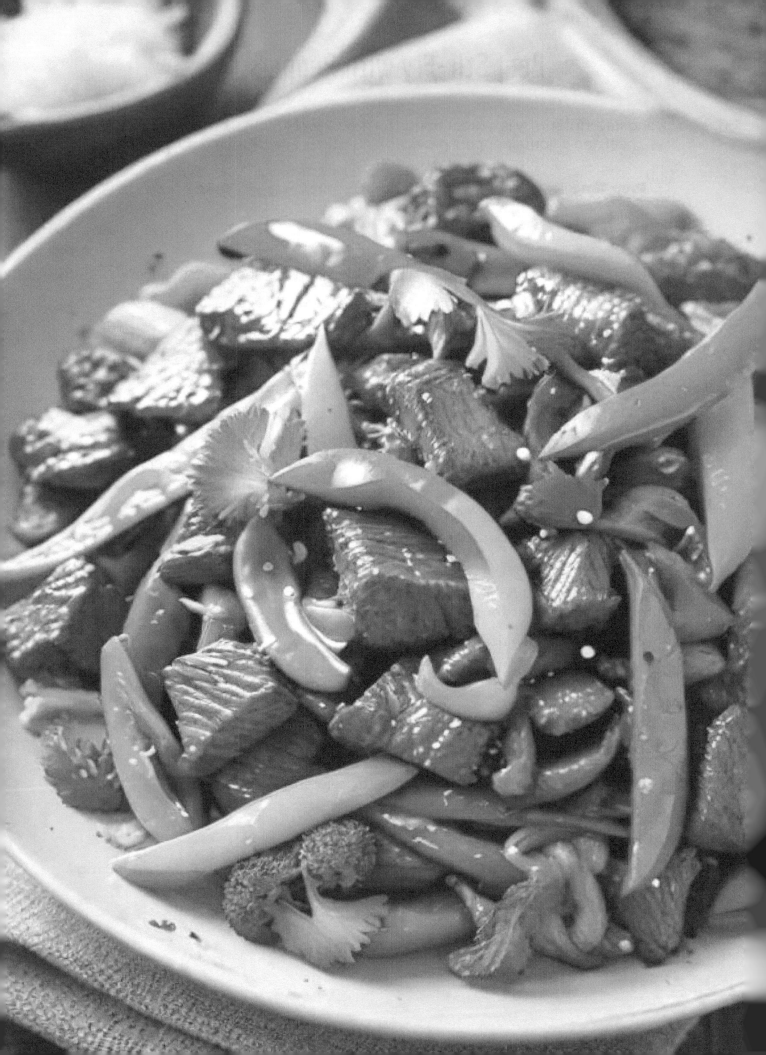

Beef Stroganoff

This classic dish has been adapted to be lower in sodium and fat, making it suitable for a diabetic and renal diet.

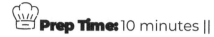 **Prep Time:** 10 minutes || 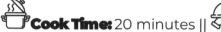 **Cook Time:** 20 minutes || 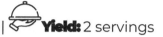 **Yield:** 2 servings

INGREDIENTS

- 8 oz lean beef tenderloin, thinly sliced
- 1/2 onion, finely chopped
- 1 clove garlic, minced
- 1 cup low-sodium beef broth
- 1/4 cup low-sodium sour cream

- 1 tablespoon Dijon mustard
- 2 tablespoons all-purpose flour
- 1/4 teaspoon dried dill
- Salt and pepper to taste
- Cooked brown rice (optional)

INSTRUCTIONS

1. In a large skillet, cook beef strips over medium-high heat until browned. Remove from skillet and set aside.

2. In the same skillet, sauté onion and garlic until softened. Sprinkle flour over the vegetables and cook for 1 minute, stirring constantly.

3. Gradually whisk in beef broth until smooth. Bring to a simmer and cook until thickened.

4. Stir in sour cream, Dijon mustard, dill, salt, and pepper.

5. Return beef to the sauce and heat through.

6. Serve over cooked brown rice, if desired.

NOTES

- For a thicker sauce, use a cornstarch slurry instead of flour.
- Serve with low-sodium noodles as an alternative to brown rice.
- You can use other lean cuts of beef, such as flank steak or round steak.

NUTRITIONAL INFO (approximate per serving):

- Calories: 250-300 | Protein: 25-30 g | Fat: 10-12 g | Carbohydrates: 15-20 g (with rice) | Sodium: 100-150 mg (may vary based on ingredients) | Potassium: 200-300 mg | Phosphorus: 100-150 mg

Hamburger Steak

This classic dish can be adapted to fit a diabetic and renal diet by using lean ground beef and limiting sodium and fat.

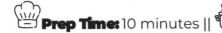 **Prep Time:** 10 minutes || 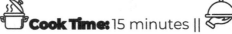 **Cook Time:** 15 minutes || 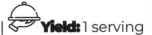 **Yield:** 1 serving

INGREDIENTS

- 4 oz lean ground beef
- 1/4 cup onion, finely chopped
- 1 clove garlic, minced
- 1/4 cup bread crumbs
- 1 egg white
- 1 tablespoon Worcestershire sauce (low sodium)
- Salt and pepper to taste
- 1 tablespoon olive oil

INSTRUCTIONS

1. In a bowl, combine ground beef, onion, garlic, bread crumbs, egg white, Worcestershire sauce, salt, and pepper. Mix well.

2. Shape the mixture into a patty.

3. Heat olive oil in a skillet over medium heat. Cook the hamburger steak for 5-7 minutes per side, or until cooked through.

4. Serve with a side of mashed cauliflower or steamed vegetables.

NOTES

- To reduce fat content, drain any excess grease from the skillet.
- Use low-sodium bread crumbs and Worcestershire sauce.
- Serve with a low-sodium gravy or mushroom sauce, if desired.

NUTRITIONAL INFO (approximate per serving):

- Calories: 250-300 | Protein: 25-30 g | Fat: 10-12 g | Carbohydrates: 5-10 g | Sodium: 100-150 mg (may vary based on ingredients) | Potassium: 200-300 mg | Phosphorus: 100-150 mg

Roasted Beef Salad

This light and refreshing salad is packed with protein and flavor, making it a perfect choice for a quick and healthy meal.

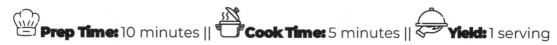 **Prep Time:** 10 minutes || **Cook Time:** 5 minutes || **Yield:** 1 serving

INGREDIENTS

- 4 oz leftover roasted beef, thinly sliced
- 1 cup mixed greens
- 1/4 cup cherry tomatoes, halved
- 1/4 cucumber, sliced
- 2 tablespoons red onion, thinly sliced
- 2 tablespoons balsamic vinaigrette (low sodium)

INSTRUCTIONS

1. In a large bowl, combine mixed greens, cherry tomatoes, cucumber, and red onion.
2. Top with thinly sliced roasted beef.
3. Drizzle with balsamic vinaigrette.
4. Serve immediately.

NOTES

- For additional flavor, consider adding a sprinkle of feta cheese or toasted almonds.
- You can adjust the amount of balsamic vinaigrette to your taste preference.
- This salad can be customized with your favorite vegetables and protein sources.

NUTRITIONAL INFO (approximate per serving):

- Calories: 200-250 | Protein: 25-30 g | Fat: 5-8 g | Carbohydrates: 5-10 g | Sodium: 100-150 mg (may vary based on ingredients) | Potassium: 200-300 mg | Phosphorus: 100-150 mg

Grilled Steak with Rice and Baked Veggies

This protein-packed meal is a balanced option for those on a diabetic and renal diet. The grilling method helps to reduce fat content.

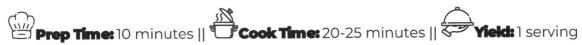 **Prep Time:** 10 minutes || **Cook Time:** 20-25 minutes || **Yield:** 1 serving

INGREDIENTS

- 4 oz lean steak (e.g., flank, sirloin)
- 1/2 cup cooked brown rice
- 1/2 cup mixed vegetables (e.g., broccoli, carrots, bell pepper)
- 1 tablespoon olive oil
- Seasonings: salt, pepper, garlic powder, onion powder

INSTRUCTIONS

1. Preheat grill to medium-high heat.

2. Season the steak with salt, pepper, garlic powder, and onion powder.

3. Grill the steak for 5-7 minutes per side, or to desired doneness. Let rest for 5 minutes before slicing.

4. While the steak is grilling, preheat oven to 400°F (200°C).

5. Toss mixed vegetables with olive oil and your preferred seasonings.

6. Spread vegetables on a baking sheet and roast for 15-20 minutes, or until tender-crisp.

7. Serve grilled steak with cooked brown rice and roasted vegetables.

NOTES

- For a quicker meal, use pre-cooked brown rice.
- Experiment with different types of vegetables based on your preference.
- To reduce sodium intake, use fresh garlic and onion instead of powdered versions.

NUTRITIONAL INFO (approximate per serving):

- Calories: 300-350 | Protein: 30-35 g | Fat: 10-12 g | Carbohydrates: 30-35 g | Sodium: 100-150 mg (may vary based on ingredients) | Potassium: 300-400 mg | Phosphorus: 150-200 mg

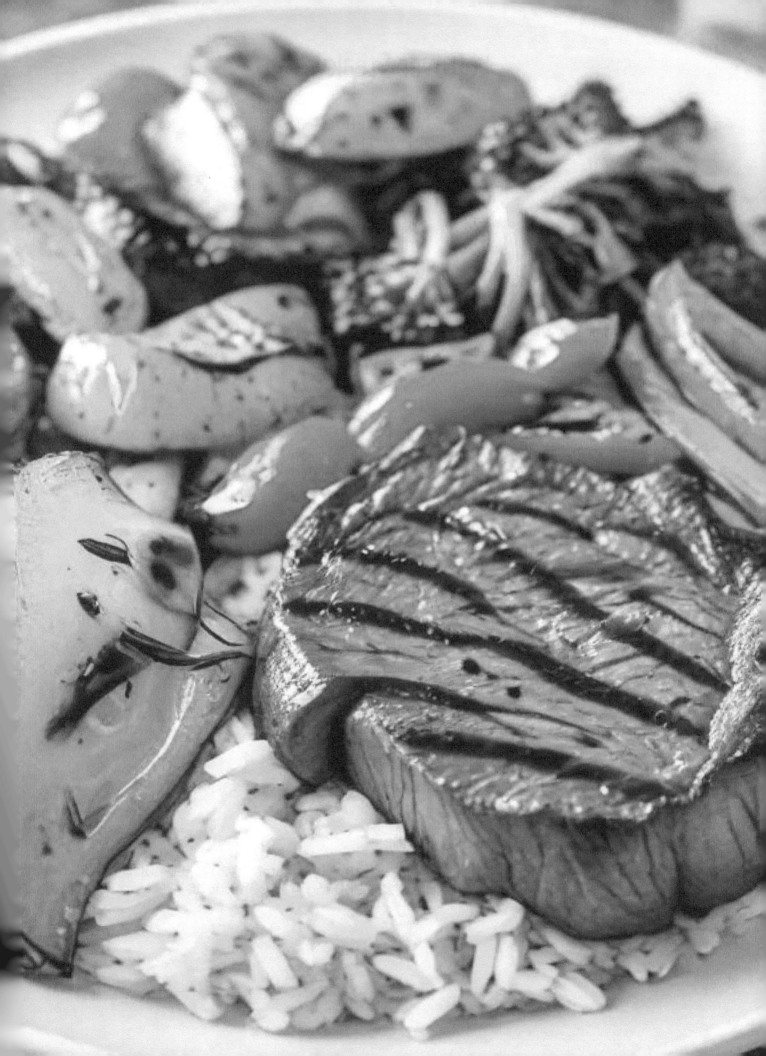

Leftover Steak Wrap

This quick and easy wrap is a great way to repurpose leftover steak while keeping within a diabetic and renal diet.

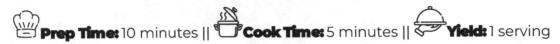 **Prep Time:** 10 minutes || **Cook Time:** 5 minutes || **Yield:** 1 serving

INGREDIENTS

- 1 leftover cooked steak, sliced into thin strips
- 1 whole-wheat or low-carb tortilla
- 1/4 cup shredded low-sodium cheddar cheese
- 1/4 avocado, sliced
- 1 tablespoon light sour cream
- 1/4 cup mixed greens
- Salt and pepper to taste

INSTRUCTIONS

1. Warm the tortilla in a skillet or microwave for a few seconds until pliable.

2. Spread a thin layer of light sour cream on the tortilla.

3. Top with sliced steak, shredded cheese, avocado, and mixed greens.

4. Season with salt and pepper to taste.

5. Fold the tortilla in half to create a wrap.

NOTES

- You can substitute other low-sodium cheeses for cheddar, such as Monterey Jack or Swiss.
- For a lower-carb option, use a lettuce wrap instead of a tortilla.
- Add your favorite low-sodium condiments, such as mustard or salsa, for extra flavor.

NUTRITIONAL INFO (approximate per serving):

- Calories: 250-300 | Protein: 25-30 g | Fat: 10-12 g | Carbohydrates: 15-20 g | Sodium: 100-150 mg (may vary based on ingredients) | Potassium: 200-300 mg | Phosphorus: 100-150 mg

CONVERSION GUIDE & MEAL PLANNERS

KITCHEN CONVERSIONS

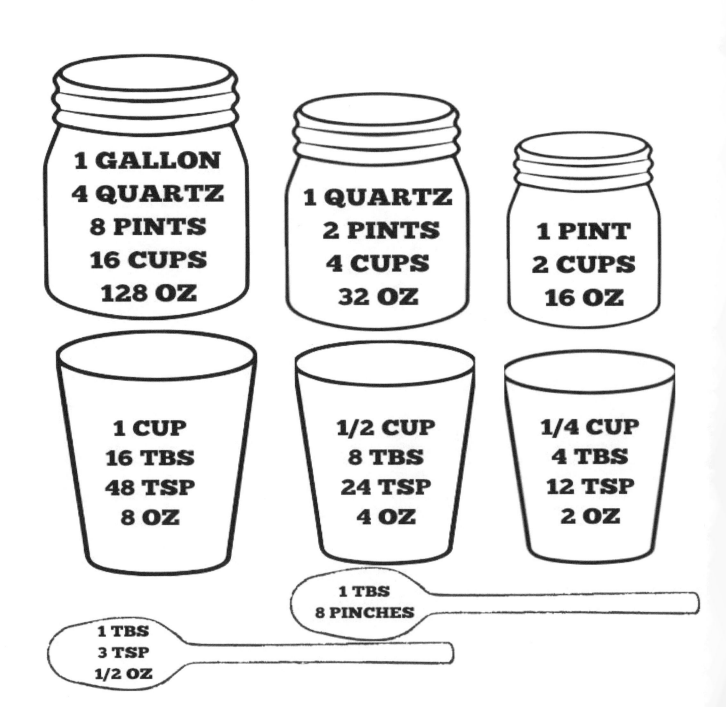

1 GALLON
4 QUARTZ
8 PINTS
16 CUPS
128 OZ

1 QUARTZ
2 PINTS
4 CUPS
32 OZ

1 PINT
2 CUPS
16 OZ

1 CUP
16 TBS
48 TSP
8 OZ

1/2 CUP
8 TBS
24 TSP
4 OZ

1/4 CUP
4 TBS
12 TSP
2 OZ

1 TBS
8 PINCHES

1 TBS
3 TSP
1/2 OZ

Dates

	BREAKFAST	LUNCH	DINNER	SNACKS
MON				
TUE				
WED				
THU				
FRI				
SAT				
SUN				

Shopping list

Dates

_____

	BREAKFAST	LUNCH	DINNER	SNACKS
MON				
TUE				
WED				
THU				
FRI				
SAT				
SUN				

Shopping list

_____ _____ _____

_____ _____ _____

_____ _____ _____

_____ _____ _____

_____ _____ _____

_____ _____ _____

Dates

	BREAKFAST	LUNCH	DINNER	SNACKS
MON				
TUE				
WED				
THU				
FRI				
SAT				
SUN				

Shopping list

_____ _____ _____
_____ _____ _____
_____ _____ _____
_____ _____ _____
_____ _____ _____

Dates

Dates
_____

	BREAKFAST	LUNCH	DINNER	SNACKS
MON				
TUE				
WED				
THU				
FRI				
SAT				
SUN				

Shopping list

_____   _____   _____

_____   _____   _____

_____   _____   _____

_____   _____   _____

_____   _____   _____

GROCERY LIST

DATE: /   /

DAIRY:
- ○ _____
- ○ _____
- ○ _____
- ○ _____
- ○ _____
- ○ _____
- ○ _____
- ○ _____
- ○ _____
- ○ _____
- ○ _____
- ○ _____

MEAT & SEAFOOD:
- ○ _____
- ○ _____
- ○ _____
- ○ _____
- ○ _____
- ○ _____
- ○ _____
- ○ _____
- ○ _____
- ○ _____
- ○ _____
- ○ _____

FRUITS & VEGGIES:
- ○ _____
- ○ _____
- ○ _____
- ○ _____
- ○ _____
- ○ _____
- ○ _____

BREAD & CEREAL:
- ○ _____
- ○ _____
- ○ _____
- ○ _____
- ○ _____

OTHERS:
- ○ _____
- ○ _____
- ○ _____
- ○ _____
- ○ _____
- ○ _____
- ○ _____

FROZEN FOODS:
- ○ _____
- ○ _____
- ○ _____
- ○ _____
- ○ _____

CANNED GOODS:
- ○ _____
- ○ _____
- ○ _____
- ○ _____
- ○ _____

WHAT'S COOKING:
- S
- M
- T
- W
- T
- F
- S

GROCERY LIST

DATE: / /

DAIRY:
- ○ _____
- ○ _____
- ○ _____
- ○ _____
- ○ _____
- ○ _____
- ○ _____
- ○ _____
- ○ _____
- ○ _____
- ○ _____
- ○ _____

MEAT & SEAFOOD:
- ○ _____
- ○ _____
- ○ _____
- ○ _____
- ○ _____
- ○ _____
- ○ _____
- ○ _____
- ○ _____
- ○ _____
- ○ _____
- ○ _____

FRUITS & VEGGIES:
- ○ _____
- ○ _____
- ○ _____
- ○ _____
- ○ _____
- ○ _____
- ○ _____
- ○ _____

BREAD & CEREAL:
- ○ _____
- ○ _____
- ○ _____
- ○ _____
- ○ _____

OTHERS:
- ○ _____
- ○ _____
- ○ _____
- ○ _____
- ○ _____
- ○ _____
- ○ _____
- ○ _____

FROZEN FOODS:
- ○ _____
- ○ _____
- ○ _____
- ○ _____
- ○ _____

CANNED GOODS:
- ○ _____
- ○ _____
- ○ _____
- ○ _____
- ○ _____

WHAT'S COOKING:
- S
- M
- T
- W
- T
- F
- S

Renal Diet Progress Diary Template

Instructions:

- Get a notebook and fill out this diary daily to keep track of your dietary intake and overall health.

- Make sure to include portion sizes and any seasonings or extras added to your meals.

- Review this diary with your healthcare provider or dietitian regularly to ensure your dietary needs are being met.

Daily Entry

Date:_____

Breakfast:

- Time:

- Foods and Beverages Consumed (include portion sizes):

- Comments (e.g., taste, any difficulty eating):

Mid-Morning Snack:

- Time:

- Foods and Beverages Consumed (include portion sizes):

- Comments:

Lunch:

- Time:

- Foods and Beverages Consumed (include portion sizes):

- Comments:

Afternoon Snack:

- Time:

- Foods and Beverages Consumed (include portion sizes):

- Comments:

Dinner:

- Time:

- Foods and Beverages Consumed (include portion sizes):

- Comments:

Evening Snack:

- Time:

- Foods and Beverages Consumed (include portion sizes):

- Comments:

Fluid Intake:

- Total Fluid Intake (in ml/oz):

- Types of Fluids Consumed:

- Comments:

Medications and Supplements:

- List of Medications and Supplements Taken:

- Time Taken:

- Comments:

Daily Health Indicators:

- Weight (in lbs/kg):

- Blood Pressure (if monitored):

- Blood Sugar Level (if monitored):

- Urine Output (if monitored, in ml/oz):

- Comments on Physical Symptoms (e.g., swelling, fatigue, nausea):

Exercise and Physical Activity:

- Type of Activity:

- Duration:

- Intensity:

- Comments:

Overall Wellness:

- Energy Levels (1-10):

- Mood (1-10):

- Any Other Comments on Well-being:

Notes for Healthcare Provider:

- Any questions or concerns for your next appointment:

- Any changes in symptoms or new symptoms experienced:

Weekly Summary

Week of [Date Range]:

Overall Diet Adherence:

- How well did you follow your renal diet this week? (1-10):

- Any challenges faced:

Fluid Management:

- Was it difficult to manage your fluid intake? (Yes/No):

- Comments:

Symptoms and Health Indicators:

- Any new symptoms or changes in existing symptoms:

- General health summary for the week:

Goals for Next Week:

- Specific dietary goals:

- Fluid intake goals:

- Health monitoring goals:

- Any other personal health goals:

This diary is designed to help you stay on track with your renal diet and manage your CKD more effectively. Remember to bring this diary to your appointments and discuss any concerns or questions with your healthcare provider.

14-Day Diabetic Renal Diet Meal Plan

This 14-day meal plan incorporates a balance of low-sodium, kidney-friendly, and diabetic-friendly meals. It provides a variety of nutrient-rich foods while carefully managing sodium, potassium, and phosphorus intake.

DAY 1

- **Breakfast:** Greek Yogurt with Berries

- **Lunch:** Quinoa Salad with Grilled Salmon and Avocado

- **Snack:** Clementines

- **Dinner:** Chicken Marsala with Steamed Green Beans and Brown Rice Pilaf

- **Dessert:** Baked Apples

DAY 2

- **Breakfast:** Scrambled Egg Whites with Spinach and Whole-Grain Toast with Almond Butter

- **Lunch:** Mediterranean Chickpea Salad

- **Snack:** Vegetable Sticks with Hummus

- **Dinner:** Baked Salmon with Asparagus

- **Dessert:** Fresh Fruit Sorbet

DAY 3

- **Breakfast:** Oatmeal with Apples

- **Lunch:** Whole-Wheat Penne with Roasted Red Pepper Pesto

- **Snack:** Rice Cakes with Low-Sodium Toppings

- **Dinner:** Chicken and Vegetable Curry

- **Dessert:** Fruit Salsa and Sweet Chips

DAY 4

- **Breakfast:** Avocado Toast

- **Lunch:** Grilled Chicken Salad

- **Snack:** Trail Mix: Three Variants

- **Dinner:** Grilled Shrimp with Zucchini

- **Dessert:** Rice Pudding

DAY 5

- **Breakfast:** Overnight Chia Seed Pudding

- **Lunch:** Lentil Loaf with Steamed Broccoli

- **Snack:** Cranberry Orange Muffins

- **Dinner:** Cajun Grilled Whitefish with Quinoa

- **Dessert:** Grilled Pineapple

DAY 6

- **Breakfast:** Protein Pancakes with Fresh Berries

- **Lunch:** Whole-Grain Couscous with Roasted Vegetables

- **Snack:** Clementines

- **Dinner:** Tarragon Chicken with Farro Salad

- **Dessert:** Fruit Crumble

DAY 7

- **Breakfast:** Breakfast Frittata

- **Lunch:** Shrimp Scampi Pasta

- **Snack:** Baked Apples

- **Dinner:** Beef Stir-Fry with Peppers and Brown Rice

- **Dessert:** Three-Grain Raspberry Muffins

DAY 8

- **Breakfast:** Protein Waffles

- **Lunch:** Turkey and Avocado Wrap

- **Snack:** Fresh Fruit Sorbet

- **Dinner:** Pan-Seared Salmon with Pineapple Salsa and Quinoa

- **Dessert:** Grilled Pineapple

DAY 9

- **Breakfast:** Cottage Cheese with Pineapple

- **Lunch:** Vegetable Stir-Fry with Tofu

- **Snack:** Fruit Salsa and Sweet Chips

- **Dinner:** Herb-Roasted Chicken Breast with Brown Rice Pilaf

- **Dessert:** Baked Apples

DAY 10

- **Breakfast:** Oatmeal with Berries and Maple Syrup

- **Lunch:** Vegetable Burger with Side Salad

- **Snack:** Rice Cakes with Low-Sodium Toppings

- **Dinner:** Poached Salmon with Dill Sauce and Green Beans

- **Dessert:** Rice Pudding

DAY 11

- **Breakfast:** Protein Smoothie

- **Lunch:** Pesto Pasta with Grilled Chicken

- **Snack:** Vegetable Sticks with Hummus

- **Dinner:** Chicken Piccata with Farro Salad

- **Dessert:** Cranberry Orange Muffins

DAY 12

- **Breakfast:** Open-Faced Egg Salad Sandwich

- **Lunch:** Mediterranean Chicken with Quinoa Salad

- **Snack:** Clementines

- **Dinner:** Grilled Shrimp with Veggies

- **Dessert:** Fresh Fruit Sorbet

DAY 13

- **Breakfast:** Avocado Smoothie

- **Lunch:** Lentil Pasta with Tomato Sauce and Vegetables

- **Snack:** Trail Mix: Three Variants

- **Dinner:** Chicken Fajitas with Whole-Grain Tortillas

- **Dessert:** Baked Apples

DAY 14

- **Breakfast:** Breakfast Burritos

- **Lunch:** Shrimp Salad with Whole-Grain Crackers

- **Snack:** Fruit Crumble

- **Dinner:** Grilled Steak with Rice and Baked Veggies

- **Dessert:** Fresh Fruit Sorbet

This meal plan is designed to provide variety and balance while being mindful of dietary restrictions for individuals managing CKD and diabetes. Always consult with a registered dietitian or healthcare provider to ensure the meal plan aligns with your specific health needs.

Exercise Plan For Individuals With Chronic Kidney Disease (Ckd) And Diabetes

This exercise plan is designed to be gentle yet effective, supporting kidney health, blood sugar management, and overall well-being. Before starting any exercise program, consult your healthcare provider to ensure it's safe for you, especially if you have any other health conditions or limitations.

Exercise Goals

- **Improve Cardiovascular Health:** Enhance heart and lung function to reduce the risk of cardiovascular disease, a common concern for those with CKD and diabetes.

- **Maintain Muscle Strength:** Prevent muscle loss and maintain physical strength, which is essential for daily activities and overall health.

- **Enhance Flexibility and Balance:** Improve flexibility and balance to reduce the risk of falls, which can be especially important as CKD progresses.

- **Manage Weight and Blood Sugar:** Support healthy weight management and improve blood sugar control through regular physical activity.

Weekly Exercise Schedule

This schedule provides a balanced mix of cardiovascular, strength, flexibility, and balance exercises. Aim to exercise most days of the week, with at least one rest day.

Monday: Cardiovascular Exercise (30-45 minutes)

- **Activity:** Brisk walking, swimming, or cycling.

- **Intensity:** Moderate. You should be able to talk but not sing during the exercise.

- **Warm-Up:** Start with 5 minutes of light walking or stretching.

- **Main Workout:** Walk at a brisk pace, swim at a comfortable speed, or cycle on a stationary bike. Aim for 30 minutes of continuous activity.

- **Cool-Down:** Finish with 5-10 minutes of slow walking and gentle stretching.

Tuesday: Strength Training (20-30 minutes)

- **Activity:** Light resistance exercises using resistance bands, dumbbells, or body weight.

- **Exercises:**

 1. **Chair Squats:** 2 sets of 10-15 reps

 2. **Bicep Curls:** 2 sets of 10-15 reps with light dumbbells or resistance bands

 3. **Wall Push-Ups:** 2 sets of 10-15 reps

 4. **Seated Leg Extensions:** 2 sets of 10-15 reps per leg

 5. **Standing Calf Raises:** 2 sets of 15-20 reps

- **Warm-Up:** 5 minutes of light cardio (marching in place or gentle walking).

- **Cool-Down:** 5 minutes of stretching, focusing on the legs and arms.

Wednesday: Flexibility and Balance (20-30 minutes)

- **Activity:** Yoga or stretching routine.

- **Exercises:**

 1. **Seated Forward Bend:** 2-3 minutes

 2. **Standing Quadriceps Stretch:** 30 seconds per leg, repeat twice

 3. **Cat-Cow Stretch (on hands and knees):** 1-2 minutes

 4. **Child's Pose:** 2-3 minutes

 5. **Standing Balance (Tree Pose):** 30 seconds per leg, repeat twice

 6. **Ankle Circles:** 10 circles in each direction per foot

- **Warm-Up:** Gentle walking or marching in place for 5 minutes.

- **Cool-Down:** Deep breathing exercises, focusing on relaxing each muscle group.

Thursday: Cardiovascular Exercise (30-45 minutes)

- **Activity:** Low-impact aerobics, dancing, or water aerobics.

- **Intensity:** Moderate.

- **Warm-Up:** 5 minutes of light movement or stretching.

- **Main Workout:** Engage in 30 minutes of continuous aerobic activity. If you enjoy dancing, put on your favorite music and dance!

- **Cool-Down:** 5-10 minutes of stretching or slow movement to bring your heart rate down.

Friday: Strength Training (20-30 minutes)

- **Activity:** Resistance exercises with a focus on different muscle groups.

- **Exercises:**

  1. **Lateral Arm Raises:** 2 sets of 10-15 reps with light dumbbells

  2. **Standing Side Leg Lifts:** 2 sets of 10-15 reps per leg

  3. **Chest Press (using resistance band):** 2 sets of 10-15 reps

  4. **Seated Row (using resistance band):** 2 sets of 10-15 reps

  5. **Glute Bridges:** 2 sets of 10-15 reps

- **Warm-Up:** 5 minutes of light cardio or dynamic stretches.

- **Cool-Down:** 5 minutes of stretching, focusing on the chest, back, and legs.

Saturday: Active Recovery (20-30 minutes)

- **Activity:** Gentle activities that promote movement without strain, such as leisurely walking, gardening, or tai chi.

- **Focus:** Relaxation and gentle movement to keep the body active without intense exertion.

- **Warm-Up:** 5 minutes of light movement.

- **Cool-Down:** Gentle stretching or deep breathing exercises.

Sunday: Rest Day

- **Activity:** Take a break from structured exercise. Focus on relaxation, mindfulness, or light activities like stretching or a gentle walk.

Tips for Success

- **Consistency is Key:** Aim to stick to the schedule, but listen to your body. If you feel tired or unwell, it's okay to take an extra rest day.

- **Stay Hydrated:** Drink water before, during, and after exercise, as recommended by your healthcare provider. Be mindful of your fluid intake if you have restrictions due to CKD.

- **Monitor Blood Sugar:** If you have diabetes, check your blood sugar levels before and after exercise, especially if you're trying a new routine or exercising at a higher intensity.

- **Use Proper Footwear:** Wear comfortable, supportive shoes to prevent foot injuries, particularly important for individuals with diabetes.

- **Incorporate Mindfulness:** End your workouts with a few minutes of deep breathing or meditation to help reduce stress and improve mental well-being.

- **Track Your Progress:** Keep a journal of your workouts, noting how you feel before and after exercise. This can help you and your healthcare team adjust the plan as needed.

Special Considerations

- **Avoid Overexertion:** Start slowly and gradually increase the intensity and duration of your workouts. Pay attention to how your body feels, and don't push yourself too hard.

- **Modify Exercises if Necessary:** If an exercise feels too challenging or causes discomfort, modify it or choose a different activity that suits your abilities.

- **Work with a Physical Therapist:** If you're new to exercise or have specific mobility issues, consider working with a physical therapist who can tailor exercises to your needs and ensure proper form.

This exercise plan is designed to be adaptable to your individual health status and fitness level, providing a comprehensive approach to managing CKD and diabetes through physical activity. By following this plan, you can improve your overall health, enhance kidney function, and enjoy a more active, fulfilling life.

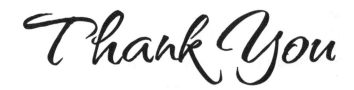

Thank You

Dear Reader,

Thank you for purchasing this cookbook. Creating this cookbook has been a labor of love, and I hope it has inspired you to explore new flavors and techniques in your kitchen. Each recipe has been crafted with care and passion, with the aim to cater to your health and diet requirements.

Your support means the world to me, and I am deeply grateful for your trust in my recipes. As you cook your way through the pages of this book, I hope you find as much joy in making these dishes as I did in creating them.

Jane Garraway

Your Feedback Matters

I would love to hear about your experiences with the recipes in this cookbook. Your honest reviews and feedback are incredibly valuable and help me continue to improve and share the joy of cooking with others. Whether it's a dish that turned out perfectly or one that you think could use some tweaking, your insights are welcomed and appreciated.

Please consider leaving a review on the platform where you purchased this book. Your feedback helps guide future books and ensures that I can continue to provide recipes that resonate with home cooks everywhere.

Thank you once again for your support.

Made in United States
Cleveland, OH
17 December 2024

12095274R00103